Many Lifetimes

OTHER BOOKS BY JOAN GRANT:

Winged Pharaoh
Eyes of Horus
Lord of the Horizon
So Moses Was Born
Return to Elysium
Life as Carola
Scarlet Feather

Far Memory

A Lot To Remember

Many Lifetimes

MANY LIFETIMES

by Joan Grant
& Denys Kelsey

with a preface by Robert R. Leichtman, M.D.

ARIEL PRESS
Atlanta, Georgia — Columbus, Ohio

First Ariel Press printing 1997

This book is made possible
by an anonymous gift
to the Publications Fund of Light

ISBN 0-89804-161-9

PREFACE

by Robert R. Leichtman, M.D.

Do we live many lives? Is our personality partly shaped by hardships and struggles from more than one life? Are some of our current problems due to the unresolved conflicts from our past lives?

I have no doubt that all of these questions can be answered with an unequivocal yes!

Reincarnation has been—and probably always will be—a controversial topic. Materialists deny anything beyond the physical, hence, even the possibility of reincarnation. Fundamentalists repudiate reincarnation because they automatically reject anything that is not part of their dogma. Skeptics do so because they enjoy ridiculing anything they haven't personally experienced.

The thinking person, however, will be delighted to read this book about reincarnation. Denys Kelsey and Joan Grant have written a volume that bypasses the theoretical basis and arguments about reincarnation in favor of *demonstrating* how exploring past lives has very practical significance. While others get bogged down in trying to justify the theory of reincarnation and how it fits into the traditions of Western religious teachings, Kelsey and Grant proceed to explore the influence of past lives on our current physical and psychological difficulties. And not only do they accomplish this, they do it with a flair and insight that is compelling in the detail and odyssey of each client described.

This book will be of great interest to those intelligent parents who are already very suspicious that their children seem to demonstrate adult qualities and insights beyond their age and meager experiences. Likewise, many competent counselors and psychotherapists will be intrigued by the possibility that the roots of their clients' difficulties may have been generated in previous lives. They will find this book helpful in finding what may be the "missing link" in comprehending the complexity of these issues.

Students of spiritual matters will find the concept of reincarnation presented in this volume very helpful in exploring the actual working out of the dynamic laws that govern right human relationships. The invisible influence of these subtle forces seems to encourage and enforce accountability for our actions—even to carrying over the resolution of unfinished obligations into future lives.

In recent years, the investigation of past lives has become a fad as common as the use of Ouija boards was a few decades ago. It is sheer luck that anything worthwhile ever comes out of those who use these things when motivated largely by curiosity and a fascination with the latest craze. Those who are unfamiliar with the limits of hypnosis—but love to use it anyway—often have little appreciation of how suggestible people become in hypnotic trance. The fantasies and fears of *both* the subject's and hypnotist's subconscious can easily "put on a show" that has little relation to fact.

In this volume, the authors present a far more effective way to explore past lives. The association of a professional psychologist (Kelsey) working with a high grade and enlightened psychic (Grant) is an unusual combination—one that fosters an effective link with

6

past life data. The presence of a competent psychic can provide a subtle psychological and psychic climate that helps the client tap into genuine past life memories. The presence of a competent psychologist and professional hypnotist helps to provide guidance and direction that avoids the evocation of irrelevant memories and the fantasy life of the client.

It is said that the real test for the usefulness of any idea or technique lies in what happens when you use it. If this is our criterion for what to believe and accept, then the authors have presented ample evidence for the fact and usefulness of reincarnation. Kelsey and Grant have given us an intriguing glimpse into the real value and applications of reincarnation. While it is impossible to verify the literal details of the past lives reported in the cases presented, it is possible to appreciate the valuable role that these past life insights played in helping these people get well again and go on to live more healthy and productive lives. These results speak loudly for the merit of their book and for validating the concept of reincarnation.

Robert R. Leichtman, M.D., is an author, teacher, and lecturer living in Baltimore, Md. A medical doctor, he focuses his abundant psychic talents on research into the fields of reincarnation, esoteric psychology, and the spiritual life. He is author of the From Heaven to Earth *series and co-author of* Active Meditation, The Art of Living, The Life of Spirit, *and* I Ching On Line, *all published by Ariel Press. Ariel Press also publishes all of the Joan Grant "far memory" novels.*

Many Lifetimes

1

FAR MEMORY

by Joan Grant

I was twenty-nine before I managed to recover the technique of being able to relive an earlier incarnation in detail and as a deliberate exercise. Until then, my conviction that I had had many lifetimes before I was born of English parents, in London, on the 12th April 1907, was based on disjointed episodes from seven previous lives, four male and three female. These episodes, although as natural as memories from more immediate yesterdays, are frustrating, because I could not fill in the gaps in continuity which would have linked them into coherent sequences.

That everyone else did not have even this small degree of far memory was so difficult to understand, that until I was eleven I presumed that other people's reticence about their own long-history was only another of the incomprehensible taboos that complicated an Edwardian childhood. I also thought that everyone else had second sight; for as grown-ups pretended not to see each other if they met while scuttling in dressing-gowns to the bathroom, it seemed no more, and no less, illogical that they pretended to ignore anyone who did not happen to be conventionally clothed in a physical body.

In my early twenties, by which time I was married to Leslie Grant and had a daughter, Gillian, I tried to extend the range of my perception by waking myself several times each night in order to write down my dreams. The majority of these dreams were only fragments of intellectual data forming patterns which had no more significance than those formed by revolving a kaleidoscope. But there were a few fertile grains among the chaff, and about twice a week I either brought back a clear recollection of what I had been doing on a supramaterial level of activity, or some incident which I knew concerned one of my earlier personalities.

By this time I had acquired sufficient empirical experience to see the broad outlines of the progress of an individual during the initial four phases of his evolution. He starts with only enough energy to organise a single molecule. As this energy increases, and his consciousness begins to expand, he requires more complex forms through which to express them. After growing too adult to be contained by the mineral phase of existence, he enters the vegetable kingdom, and then graduates, by a series of incarnations as various species of animal, to his first incarnation as a member of the race of Homo sapiens.

During his first few lifetimes as a human-being the whole of his personality incarnates, so he is likely to have approximately the same capacities and perceptions whether he happens to be incarnate or excarnate. But as his consciousness expands it becomes too wide to be contained within the framework of a single per-sonality. So the incarnate individual is now both a single personality and an integral component of his total self. He is in effect both the segment of an orange and part of the whole orange: the juice, which is the essence of them both, being the character he has acquired by his own efforts during the course of his personal evolution.

Having been educated less through the efforts of numerous governesses and tutors than by listening to the conversation of my father and his fellow scientists, and then working for four years as a laboratory assistant in his Mosquito Control Institute, I was always alert to the possibility that the incidents of far memory might be only fantasies based on my hopes and fears, or on what I had heard or seen or read. Had radio, television, or more than a primitive form of cinematograph then been invented, my self-doubts would have been even more acute.

With practise I eventually learned how to discriminate between the pseudo and the factual, between a thought-form I had created, such as the thought-forms of the position of chessmen when playing the game without looking at the board, and a scene which had its own objective reality. To take a simple example: if I saw two men walking across a courtyard, one wearing a red and the other a green tunic, and I could change the colour of the tunics, or even turn the tunics into kilts, then it was only a thought-form. If the scene could not be altered, however intently I tried to change it, then I accepted its validity.

A more personally convincing check was that the emotions and the sensations associated with a genuine recall were as vivid as though they were being felt by myself in the factual present. The alteration of the focus of my attention had caused an incident in the past again to become Here and Now. Sometimes this could be not only terrifying but physically painful, for there was no awareness of the intervening period of clock time to cushion the immediacy of the impact.

So far as I have been able to discover, it is no more difficult to recall an episode which took place several millennia ago than to recall one from the current or the preceding century. Here the analogy between a series of personalities and the segments of an orange is again apposite, time being the centre at which the segments join and from which they are equidistant. The concept of successive personalities being threaded by Time like beads on a string is intellectually expedient but misleading.

Experience suggests that the earlier life which has the greatest resonance to the current one is the most likely to be recalled. This resonance may be set in motion by some close similarity of situation, by some mutual direction of effort, or by a resurgence of intense emotion. Revisiting a once familiar scene can sometimes evoke a spontaneous flashback, but this is seldom of more than mild interest. I spent three weeks in Egypt, with Leslie in March 1935, but except for being surprised that certain avenues of trees no longer led from Hat-shep-sut's temple to Karnak, and feeling depressed that there were so many ruins instead of being pleased that there was so much left to see, I had no intimations that I had spent the best part of two thousand years in the Nile Valley.

Eighteen months later, through the trivial catalyst of psychometrising a scarab, I did the first of the 115 total recalls which became a posthumous autobiography of over 120,000 words. The scarab belonged to Daisy Sartorius, whose house had become my real home since the day I went there during a particularly unhappy crisis of my youth. She had already had the first of several operations for the cancer from which she died a year later, and it was the love we shared which caused me to concentrate on a life in which she had been my mother in the first Dynasty of Egypt, about 3000 years B.C.

The technique of this type of far-memory, as opposed to the isolated incident which is a spontaneous recall or recovered with the aid of hypnosis, entails learning how to shift the level of the majority of one's attention from the current personality to the earlier one, while still retaining sufficient normal waking consciousness to dictate a running commentary of the

earlier personality's thoughts, emotions, and sensations. During the early stages I would often think I had
been dictating clearly, only to discover at the end of a
session that I had not spoken a word. On other occasions I would think I had been speaking so slowly that
at least a minute had elapsed between each phrase:
and then find that I had been talking so fast that Leslie,
who could do Speedwriting but not shorthand, had
been able to get down only a bare outline of what I had
said. Eventually I was to accept an instruction to speak
louder or more slowly, but this took considerable practice, and until I had gained it, any kind of interruption
would break the thread of concentration and I might
not be able to get anything at all for two or three days.

Although I would usually begin a session by giving
the age of Sekeeta—which was that earlier personality's
name, I could not predetermine which period of her
life I was going to relive. One session might find me
enjoying some happy incident from her childhood
and in the next she was watching an operation in
which a man's skull was being trepanned after he had
been thrown from his chariot during a lion hunt. By
this time I knew that Sekeeta was the daughter of
Pharaoh and that she became co-ruler with her brother
after her father's death.

Between an idyllic childhood and the lonely years of
rulership Sekeeta spent ten years in a temple learning
the far-memory which would allow her to speak with
personal authority. The temples of that time were not
places of worship but were comparable to co-educa-
tional universities or teaching hospitals in which pupils learned various forms of extra-sensory perception.
Seers, whose role was similar to the modern radiolo-
gist; healers, who supplied extra energy to the physical
body of their patients and who were considered senior
to the physicians; hypnotists, who induced anæsthesia
during surgical operations or for a difficult childbirth;
and temple-counsellors, who had a great deal more

insight than the majority of modern psychiatrists—in fact they would have been amazed that the people whose label means "Healer of the soul" often do not believe in the existence of the organ they purport to treat.

Those who were training for a degree in far-memory usually gained the additional qualification of being able to tune in to the relevant episode from a patient's earlier life which was affecting his present personality. They also had to be able to remember at least ten of their own deaths so as to be able to reassure anyone who suffered from a fear of dying; although this was seldom necessary in that enlightened culture in which birth and death were familiar changes of state, as commonplace as sleeping and waking.

The graduation examination for far-memory was arduous. The pupil was shut in an initiation chamber entered by a narrow passage closed by three dropstones to increase its resemblance to a tomb, for the initiation symbolised a rebirth.

When I or rather Sekeeta heard those dropstones fall, I knew that I would be alone in the dark silence for four days and four nights. I had three alternatives. I could try to avoid the issue by staying awake, in which case I should have to leave the temple and would never be able to serve Egypt as a Winged Pharaoh, a priest as well as a ruler. I could try to do what was expected of me, and fail, which might drive me insane. . . . "Shall I be as Hekket who failed yet did not die, and who sits in the courtyard with blind eyes and wet sagging lips?" Or I must prove that I could remember other levels of reality, remember the Beautiful Country,which makes living in three dimensions seem so heavy, so small, and so drab. And remember the hells which men create for themselves, in spite of the best endeavours of their forerunners, from the substances of their own cruelty, their own paucity of affection.

Sekeeta then had to undergo seven ordeals, which

had been designed by her instructors to assure them that her insight would not be impaired by unresolved terrors from her long-history.

The recall of these four days and nights took five hours of clock-time. By then Leslie had writer's cramp and I was so exhausted that I could only drag myself upstairs by clutching the bannisters. I hoped to sleep for hours, but the Seventh Ordeal, in which Sekeeta had to overcome a gigantic cobra, had produced such a keen resurgence of my fear of snakes that within a few minutes I woke, reliving the same sequence....

"I saw before me a great pit, and islanded in a rustling sea of snakes a mighty cobra reared upon its coils. Vipers writhed and slithered across the floor, waving an endless pattern of venomed death. Yet must I walk across their chaining coils and crush the cobra between my hands. Its eyes glittered scarlet, and its mighty hood shone with the brilliance of its armoured scales. It seemed that for an endless span of time I stood with horror naked in my eyes. Then I walked into this hissing pit, and the vipers drew back before me in vicious waves. And then I seized the cobra below its swaying head and held it from me as it tried to strike.

"Ten thousand times, again ten thousand times, I thought that I had reached the final refuge of my desperate will. It seemed that time was endless and Earth grown cold, until under the last onslaught of my will the mighty serpent slid down on its coils. And I was with its dead body in an empty pit."

I was so convinced that the cobra was in the bed that Leslie, who was almost as tired as I was, could calm me only by stripping off the bedclothes and shaking them out the window. As we were then living near Grantown and it was mid-winter, when the bedroom was so cold that the water-pitcher had usually frozen solid before dawn, this was yet another occasion when I have inadvertently proved a tiresome companion. Even then I dared not sleep, and had rigors, cramps, fever,

16

and a blinding headache which immobilised me for forty-eight hours. Had I not known that Daisy looked forward to the copies of the sessions I posted to her nearly every day, I think that at this point I would have chosen a less exacting profession.

By now I had recorded about two hundred episodes—for a single session might include two or three incidents which apparently were entirely unrelated. At least once an hour I had to break concentration for a brief rest, and often was then unable to tune in to the same sequence. If Leslie read back what I had dictated immediately I had returned to normal waking-consciousness, I could supply a word he had missed, but after about ten minutes the memory had faded and I could remember no more than a hazy outline of what I had been saying. I wish tape recorders had already been available because I have often been told that the emotional colour of my voice, which is normally very flat, had a remarkably wide range; but during this type of level-shift it sounds to me remote and impersonal, so this is only hearsay.

One day Leslie and I spread all the episodes out on the drawing-room floor to arrange them in chronological sequence. For the first time I noticed that two parts of the same conversation often dovetailed completely, even though several weeks had elapsed between the two recordings. For instance, a session which began, "When I was twenty-three..." concerned a long conversation with someone called Ptah-kefer, which was interrupted by the insistent ringing of the telephone. When Leslie asked, "This is the first time Ptah-kefer has been mentioned: who is he?" I could not tell him, for I was unable to shift level again that evening. For at least in my experience, far-memory entails a very precise focus of attention and, as when using a long-range telescope, the field of vision does not include anything extraneous. A few days later, when tuned in to Sekeeta's childhood, I said, "Ptah-kefer, who was one of the chief

17

officials of the Royal Household, sat on the left side of the Hall of Audience, between the throne of Pharaoh and the table of the scribes." Then, several weeks later, the first, not the second part of the conversation with Ptah-kefer was recorded, and when joined together there was not even a phrase missing in the continuity.

This was very reassuring to me, for my father's insistence on the scientific approach had made me somewhat over-sceptical of my own faculties. I knew that if I had wished to become a historical novelist I would not have been so idiotic as to make the job infinitely more complicated by inventing disjointed episodes and then hoping that they would fit like the pieces of a jigsaw puzzle. I knew that my knowledge of Egyptian history was minimal, and that if I had been venal enough to want to perpetrate an elaborate hoax I would have first embarked on a very careful historical research, instead of scrupulously not doing any. I knew that when I felt that some incident of Sekeeta's life had only one logical outcome, recall would often reveal that the facts were entirely different, neither what she would have hoped nor what I would have imagined. But I also knew that convincing as these factors were to me, they would not be accepted as evidence to anyone else.

It is unlikely that Seeketa's autobiography would ever have had a wider readership than Daisy and a few intimate friends, who were tolerant of my E.S.P. because the rest of my behaviour was so stalwartly ordinary, if, in June 1937, I had not gone to London for a wedding at which Gillian was to be a bridesmaid and Leslie the best man. While Leslie was at the groom's stag-party I dined with Guy McCaw, a contemporary of my father, whom I met by chance at Prince's Tennis Club: Royal, not lawn tennis, a game played in New York at the Racquet and Tennis Club, which I began to learn at the age of seven in my father's court.

Guy asked me, "What on earth are you doing buried up in Scotland? You can't even shoot grouse in the winter. Or have you become addicted to salmon fishing?"

Mildly annoyed that he thought no one could enjoy Scotland unless they were killing something, I forgot that I had promised Leslie to be discreet. "I catch an occasional trout when I am not too busy, but I spend most of my time remembering who I used to be when I lived in Egypt during the first Dynasty."

"Good God, Joan! Have you gone off your head?" He scrutinised me and seemed relieved that I laughed at him. "You gave me quite a shock. I didn't realise you were joking."

"I'm not joking. I have dictated about sixty thousand words of what, even if you think I made it up, is an interesting story."

"Well, let me read it." He plumed his impeccable white moustache with the back of his hand and then said pontifically, "I will read it, providing it is typed, but I am not going to wade through pages of your handwriting. I always tell people the truth, however unpalatable; so if it is nonsense I shall be brutally candid."

I had had no intention of showing anyone the carbon copy of the typescript which I had brought with me to give to Daisy. But Guy's bland assumption that any claim to far-memory could be no more than an imaginative outpouring which should be sterilised by a swab of criticism caused me to send it to him the following morning. I enclosed a brief note, thanking him for an excellent dinner and asking him to forward the typescript to Daisy, as by the time he had finished reading it I would have returned to Scotland.

I did not mention this breach of confidence to Leslie because I expected to hear nothing more about it. But Guy wrote to me, "To my great surprise you have written something far better than you apparently recognize. I consider it should be published, and have therefore given it to Arthur Barker."

Both Leslie and I were dismayed, though for different reasons: Leslie because Arthur was a fellow Wykemist, and might mention in the clubs to which they both belonged that Mrs. Grant had ideas which were exceedingly odd: I because Arthur seemed such a die-hard materialist that I thought he would throw a couple of hundred carefully typed pages into the waste-paper basket.

In fact Arthur sent me a telegram. When Leslie brought it to me—it had come over the telephone while I was out for a walk with Gillian, he looked so glum that I thought Daisy had died. It read, "Essential you complete manuscript in six weeks so that we can publish in October. Stop. Blurb will state most exciting and important book we have ever published. Stop. Congratulations. Stop. Arthur."

This telegram, although I did not recognize it at the time, heralded the termination of my first marriage.

I first became aware of the existence of the personality who became the "I" of my second book while still recording Sekeeta. Sir Henry Wood, who took it for granted that musical genius was the result of several lifetimes directed towards developing this particular talent, had been listening to me dictate. At the end of the session Leslie switched on the radio, as I had asked him to do when anyone else was present so as to spare me having to talk during the awkward period of transition between two levels. The broadcast was of Haydn, played on a harpsichord, and I mentioned that I had been listening to Egyptian music only a few minutes earlier. Henry said eagerly, "Can you hear the Egyptian music and the Haydn at the same time? For it would be very interesting if you could tell me how closely they are related."

I shifted level again very easily, and the harpsichord

went out of hearing. When I came back Leslie asked, "Can you remember where you have been and what instrument you were playing?"

I could still feel strings rippling under my fingers. "It was a lute. Which is odd because I didn't know that Egyptians had lutes. Or that Sekeeta could play any kind of musical instrument."

"You were not in Egypt but in Italy," said Leslie. "You were born near Perugia early in the sixteenth century. Don't try to talk. Wait until I have read it back to you:

"I was born early in the morning of the fourth of May, in the year of our Lord 1510, and I died in the autumn of 1537. Though I was conceived in the great bed, I opened my new eyes in the north-west turret of the House of the Griffin...my cradle was of dark, carved wood, and my mother used to rock it with her foot while she laid her silk threads into smooth stitches...she was a sewing woman of the castle. My name was Carola...my grandmother banished us when I was seven years old...before my father brought a bride from Spain. We were befriended by the strong-man of a troupe of strolling players...I learned to sing and play a lute. There was another singer and a jester—a hunchback whom I loved very much. Then something terrible happened...I can't remember yet what it was. I was in a convent. The first abbess was kind, but the next one tortured me as a heretic...but I managed to escape. I thought I was dying, but I was taken into the house of a wise and gentle old man, Carlos, who married me, and my name was Carola di Ludovici. Then he died, and I soon began to cough, and became thinner, and thinner. I was looked after by Anna...it seems that I am already separate from my body. It is not Carola whose hair Anna braids, nor Carola who drinks cordials to please her Anna. It is as though I watch her try to mend my dress and wonder why she weeps to see the velvet threadbare when I know I have to wear it so short a while....'"

In about two hundred words, dictated during twenty-five minutes, I had brought back the outline of a life which took me over two hundred sessions to record in detail.

I think the reason why Henry's question about the relationship between Haydn and Egyptian music caused me to tune in to Carola, a personality which until then I had not even glimpsed, rather than to Sekeeta, was that the sound of the harpsichord was the thread I was following while I was shifting level. A harpsichord has a closer affinity with a sixteenth-century lute than with any stringed instruments which Sekeeta had heard. Sekeeta was not particularly musical, but a lute was associated with both the happy and the harsh periods of Carola's lifetime, and for fifteen years was her only means of survival.

This session was also unique in my experience because I not only got the outline of Carola's story, but also her birth-date and her surname. The significance of dates and surnames is usually so ephemeral that they are seldom registered on the permanent components of a personality. But to Carola the date of her birth was important, because it was this which caused her father to acknowledge her as his child; and being a bastard, she had had no surname until she married. She remembered the calendar year of her death because Anna, trying to encourage her to live, so often said, "You are only twenty-seven, and far too young to die."

The last chapter of Carola's life was dictated to Charles Beatty, with whom I eloped two months earlier, just before the outbreak of World War Two. We were driving along a country road in Sussex when I suddenly had a hunch to shift level. So Charles stopped the car, and during the next three hours, lying on pine-needles in a small wood, I dictated over four thousand words. After sitting up most of the night to type them, we posted the manuscript off to Methuen the following morning.

During the next four months Charles was at the Staff College, doing the "short war course" on which everyone was trying to absorb so much condensed information that he and the other four members of his syndicate were glad that I could do their typing for them. Having no knowledge of military matters, I was surprised to find how easily I could understand problems which concerned moving troops from one sector to another and keeping them supplied at each stage with everything they needed. But I did not begin to discover the reason for this small expertise until in 1941, when Charles had been invalided out of the Army and we were living on his family estate, Trelydan, in North Wales.

I then began to record a life in which I had been the Nomarch of the Oryx, nearly a thousand years after Sekeeta. Egypt was then divided into eighteen Nomes, and a Nomarch was comparable to the Lord Lieutenant of an English county, although his authority was much wider. My name was Ra-ab Hotep: the tombs of his family, as I have since learned although I have not had a chance to visit them, are at Beni Hasan. As I remembered more about him I realised why the work I had done while Charles was at the Staff College had seemed so familiar. Ra-ab Hotep had learned how to cope with very similar problems: for if he had failed to provide sufficient water-carriers for a desert march the men he led would have been halted even more finally than an Army whose vehicles had run out of gasoline; and if the wooden hafts were the wrong diameter to fit the holes in the stone maceheads—this type of mace was flung rather than used as a club—it would have been as disconcerting as if a contemporary commander found that the ammunition for his artillery was of the wrong calibre.

During the last reign of the Eleventh Dynasty, Egypt was in decadence. Temples were no longer training-places where pupils learned the perception which qualified them to serve the community as priests, but instead were staffed by men who, in spite of their office, were effective only as collectors of tribute. The majority of the population had become so deluded that they even accepted the notion that the gods were so vain and insecure that they depended on audience-reaction and relished being worshipped.

Ra-ab Hotep belonged to a resistance movement which, although vastly outnumbered, contained enough sane individuals to overthrow a rule based on terrorisation. They were called the Eyes of Horus, a title they had adopted to remind themselves that the man of true insight must keep both his eyes open: with one he will see the gods, and with the other, the maggots in the belly of a dead crocodile. Their password was "Send Fear into Exile." If they had belonged to the present century they might have taken "Down with One-upmanship" as a slogan equally urgent and apposite.

When the Pharaoh they had chosen, Amenemhet, was proclaimed, he made a speech to the thousands who had assembled to welcome him which, although it is too long to quote in full, contains passages which I believe are worth remembering.

"I shall never forget that day; Amenemhet looked remote as a god-statue, his face under the White Crown calm as the crossed hands which held the Crook, with which he had vowed to shepherd his people, and the Flail, by which he would protect them from their enemies. Yet to each of the multitude who heard his voice he spoke as a friend, and as the link between them and their forerunners.

" 'Strive for happiness as lesser men strive for power: and remember that love is both the seed and the flower of joy. Let your actions be such that if they were done to you they would increase your happiness. Love others that they may love you: and love yourself that you may love others.

" 'This is the First Law: the imperishable rock on

24

which the New Egypt must be built. If this law be kept there will be no need for other laws; yet so that you may know what the first Law shall give you, I will tell you what harvest will spring from that single furrow if you are wise husbandmen.

"'You will be born without fear: for your mother and your father will rejoice in their fertility.

"'You will learn the speech of kindliness: so that the rasp of anger and the sound, harsh as splintered bones, of quarrels, shall be as a foreign language which holds no meaning for you.

"'Your work shall be according to the needs of your soul: though you were born in the house of a fisherman, you may become a scribe; though you are born in the house of a potter, you may become a warrior; or from the house of a field-worker you may become a noble. You shall be measured according to the weighing of your heart; neither being wearied by a field too large for you to till, nor restricted by boundaries that are too narrow.

"'You are bound to no one save by the gold link of affection. Should brother and brother be kinsmen only by blood, then will they say "Farewell" with the usages of courtesy and take different roads, rather than travel together in hostility.'"

Amenemhet then reminded them that they must guard themselves against Set, who epitomised the devolutionary aspects of mankind, envy, jealousy, and hatred.

"'You must remember always that Set may come to your door in disguise. He may offer you gold which is not yours by right. He may offer you the rod of authority when you know it is too heavy for your hand. He may offer you the strong wine of flattery which you know you are not old enough to drink. You must recognise him as your enemy; and if he will not leave you when you bid him go, then you must call upon your friends to help you drive him again into exile.

"'In obeying the first Law, you will have broken many of the arrows in Set's quiver:

"'You will not fear solitude, for you will never be friendless.

"'You will not fear your husband or your wife, for you will have taken them in love and not for expediency.

"'You will not fear your child, for no enemy can be born of love.

"'You will not fear idleness, for all are needed in the New Egypt.

"'You will not fear work, for it will be congenial.

"'You will not fear famine, for in the granaries there will be bread for the lean years.

"'You will not fear floods, for the water channels shall be maintained, and the aqueducts mighty in their cubits.

"'You will not fear to grow up, for the years will show you new horizons.

"'You will not fear to grow old, for in each horizon you will find further wisdom.

"'You will not fear death, for you shall remember the other side of the Great River.

"'You will not fear Set, but conquer him by the love in your own heart.'"

Amenemhet's promise to his people came true, and endured for more than three centuries, until the ethics of which he had reminded them were again forgotten.

During that interlude of peace and sanity I was born at lease twice in the Nile Valley, but both lives were so happy and uneventful that they are a source of nostalgia but not of a book. These gentle memories make it increasingly difficult to understand why people of our generation do not demand the same qualities of insight and integrity from their leaders. If they did so, then the leaders would be able to promise them opportunities more congenial than the prospect of being incarnated in bodies which will be less pretty, less

26

nimble, than those they are now using: for evidence suggests that none of the species on this planet will be improved by the mutations caused by radioactivity.

Ra-ab Hotep's life was published as *Eyes of Horus* and *Lord of the Horizon* in 1942 and 1943. For even after I had cut five chapters, which concerned his son and were redundant to the autobiography, the recording still ran to over a quarter of a million words, which was impractical for a single book during the wartime paper restrictions. I also cut six traditional stories which had been told to Ra-ab Hotep during his childhood and which he told to his sons and daughter: but these were spared from the bonfire and became *The Scarlet Fish.*

Recalling these stories was astoundingly easy, possibly because he had heard them while still young enough to see them as a series of vivid mental images. They may also have remained so clearly delineated because I had been told them in at least four Egyptian childhoods; and to be reminded of something one already knows always makes a more lively impression than the cautious sniff at a new piece of information. I incidentally discovered why I had always been attracted by the blue faience hippopotamuses which are in nearly every collection of Egyptian antiquities: for they illustrate the story in which a blue faience hippopotamus, who was the toy of a little princess, learned to love her so much that a kindly magician turned him into a human being so that he could be born to her and the prince she loved—the prince of whom he had managed never to be jealous.

The children at Trelydan were also the impetus which caused me to recall legends from a North American incarnation which must have been in the second millennium B.C., if as I think, it was after Sekeeta and before Ra-ab Hotep. These legends became *Redskin Morning.* The autobiography was called *Scarlet Feather,* for although I was then female I gained the right to wear a feather of this color through undergoing the ordeals required of the tribal warriors.

This life was primarily concerned with the need for men and women to resolve their conventional antagonism by recognising that they had gained their experience in both male and female bodies. The total self is androgyne, and if a personality tries to deny the instincts and intuition which were acquired while incarnate as the opposite sex, this will result in a psychological civil war, which will limit the potentialities of the individual and probably lead him or her into the social difficulties which nowadays exacerbate the problems of sexual anomaly.

The ethics of the tribe to which I belonged were condensed into a single concept. They believed that there was only one question which they would be asked by the Great Hunters before they could enter heaven, "How many people are happier because you were born?" This explicit simplicity showed that they had retained an insight into the fundamental principles of individual evolution which was closer to the original pattern even than that still held in early Egypt, where the same ideas were already becoming blurred through being more elaborately expressed as the Laws of the Forty-Two Assessors; laws which in another few centuries became the whisps of reality obscured by superstition which have survived in innumerable copies of the Book of the Dead.

During this period I was lucky if I could spare a couple of hours a day for far-memory recordings, which, because Charles was occupied with his own writing and research, I usually dictated to Kathleen Barker. After Arthur was taken prisoner at the fall of Hong Kong, Kathleen had come to live at Trelydan with their three sons. Both she and I were busy with more immediate demands on our time, for there were seldom less than ten and sometimes twenty other people sharing our roof; some of these we had known before they arrived, others became friends after landing unexpectedly on the doorstep.

Many of them needed only sleep, food, and warmth, to renew their energies for another round of the conflict. Others came because a problem which might never have come into their normal-waking-consciousness under ordinary conditions had become urgent through war strain. They required high-speed psychotherapy which often involved tuning in to the source of a specific fear which, because they had not realised it belonged to their past, they had presumed to be a premonition of their future. It was very rewarding to find that when the real origin of an acute apprehension of a particular type of death or injury, for instance drowning, burning, being crushed under falling masonry or disembowelled, had been seen by me and recognized as valid by the person who suffered from it, the fear dispersed and thereafter was no more than a normal dislike of this particular hazard.

Apart from the chores which occur when running a fairly large household, chores that in wartime extended to such items as converting an enormous dead pig into hams, bacon, sausages, a bladder of lard and other edible commodities, including three basins of brawn from every morsel of its head—which entailed tweaking the hairs out of its ears with my eyebrow tweezers, there was plenty of nursing. Luckily I had already had considerable practise in this art, for ever since I first married and had a home instead of living under the "parental roof," there were nearly always people in it who were convalescing from operations or accidents, or being cossetted through ailments ranging from pneumonia to D.T.'s.

I have always been fortunate in having sympathetic friends among doctors, so there was never any difficulty in getting expert medical assistance for the physical problems of the people I was trying to help. In fact there were several occasions when my insistence on a thorough medical checkup revealed that the real cause of a symptom, for which the patient had been undergoing psychoanalysis for months or even years, was a massive uterine fibroid rather than frigidity, or adenoids, rather than asthma caused by maternal rejection. It seemed obvious even during my adolescence, as it still does, that any divergence from the natural pattern of health or sanity should be dealt with on the level which is most appropriate. In my view, it would be as idiotic to try to remove a bullet with psychotherapy as it is to expect to cure a neurosis by numbing the patient with pills.

My unconventional approach to psychotherapy has always seemed as natural as second-sight or far-memory. I presumed this stemmed from Egyptian incarnations until, in 1945, I began to record *Return to Elysium*. I was born in Greece towards the end of the second century B.C.; my name was Lucina, and I was the ward and pupil of a philosopher who, on his estate near Athens, tried to cure patients by convincing them that sanity consisted in accepting that they had no hope of immortality.

Lucina had retained sufficient far-memory to know that this was nonsense, and eventually, after undergoing many "scientific" tests, was able to convince her guardian to whom she was devoted, that there was a fundamental flaw in his cherished premise. Instead of being glad of this insight he became distraught; so Lucina went to Rome and established a flourishing, if somewhat discreditable practice, on an island in the Tiber.

For various reasons, which are not relevant to the subject of reincarnation, I published only one other far-memory autobiography, *So Moses Was Born*, when I was a male contemporary of Rameses II. And until I met Denys in 1958, I had little opportunity to make further practical use of my conviction that in the Expanding Universe the individual also expands.

2

RECOGNITION OF A REALITY

by Denys Kelsey

I should like people to share my belief in reincarnation: I think it would cause them to be much happier, much less frightened, and very much more sane. For a psychiatrist to hold this belief and to have made it the basis of his therapy, is still rather unusual. It is not a belief which I have always held, so I will begin by explaining how I was led to it through clinical evidence which had been accumulating during the ten years before I learned that somebody called Joan Grant was able to remember many of her earlier lives. Without this work, I would not have been able so rapidly to appreciate the value of what Joan was able to contribute; because, like so many people, I cannot accept a concept unless it satisfies my intellect and relates to my empirical experience.

I was precipitated into the practice of psychiatry, at the age of thirty-one, without even an hour's warning. In this I was fortunate; it meant that I approached the subject without any preconceived ideas, for when I was a medical student, psychiatry played only a very small part in the curriculum. I remember being taught that the causes of thyrotoxicosis were "sex, sepsis, and psychic trauma;" and I attended a series of lecture-demonstrations, but rather lightheartedly because questions on psychiatry never occurred in the examinations. And that, to the best of my recollection, was that!

But immediately after embarking upon psychiatry, a series of cases came my way which, step by step, extended the framework of what I believed to be fact until, after four years, a session with a particular patient forced me to the intellectual certainty that in a human being there is a component which is not physical. To be taught this as a matter of dogma or doctrine is one thing; to be compelled to the same conclusion by one's own experiences is quite another. I did not realise it at the time, but this session was an important landmark on the way to a belief in reincarnation; at least I had got as far as believing in the reality of something which could reincarnate!

In 1948 I was working on the medical side of a large military hospital, a post which I owed to the fact that three years previously I had passed the post-graduate examination which is the start of the long road to recognition as a consulting physician or internist. I was still travelling this road when an epidemic of influenza hit the hospital and abruptly changed my course. One of the first casualties was a medical officer in the psychiatric wing and I was asked, temporarily, to take over as much of his work as I could. Late that night, I learned that I had an aptitude for inducing hypnosis.

I was summoned urgently to the ward to give a sedative injection to a patient who had suddenly become acutely disturbed and violent. By the time I arrived, three muscular orderlies had the situation under control and were holding the patient firmly down on his bed. I had a feeling that he was unlikely to resume his violence, so I motioned to the orderlies to leave. But the patient was obviously still very frightened, and with no intention beyond trying to calm his fears, I sat down beside him and began to talk to him in what I hoped was a soothing and reassuring voice. I certainly did not realise that I then began to use one of the standard techniques for inducing hypnosis. It had simply occurred to me that if I could get him to fix his attention on something outside himself he might be less disturbed by his ideas and feelings, so I asked him to fix his gaze on a dim light in the ceiling above his head. For the same reason I coaxed him to concentrate upon his breathing, making it perfectly regular and rhythmical, but a little slower and a little deeper than usual.

He was still very tense. His fists were tightly clenched and his arms and legs showed a fine tremor. So I drew his attention to each of his limbs in turn, urging him to relax them and to allow them to remain relaxed. These instructions were interspersed with reassurances that he had nothing to fight, nothing to fear. Gradually he became perceptibly calmer, until he was lying completely relaxed. Purely for good measure I continued talking to him in the same strain, and I recall suggesting to him, quite casually, that he might as well go off to sleep. At this, his eyes rolled up and his eyelids came down in a curiously positive way, and I suddenly realised to my astonishment that I must have hypnotised him!

The next morning I described the incident to the psychiatrist in charge of the department, who confirmed that this was almost certainly what had happened. He was intrigued as I, and asked me to repeat the technique on another patient, a man who was suffering from a neurosis as a result of a horrific accident with an automobile. This patient entered hypnosis very quickly, and with a tremendous release of emotion, relived the circumstances of the accident. The psychiatrist assured me that it would now be a simple matter to clear up the residue of the neurosis. During the next few weeks I was able to treat several other patients in a similar way; they too relived the relevant episodes with great release of emotion and went on to a rapid recovery. I found these experiences in the military hospital so rewarding that I decided henceforth to specialise in psychiatry. Once back in civil life I took a post in a mental hospital where I remained for the next six years.

Hypnosis has played such a large part in the experiences I shall shortly describe that I will say something about it. A convenient starting point is the widely accepted concept that there are three distinct compartments of mental activity. First, there is the compartment of consciousness, to which I shall usually refer as "normal-waking-consciousness." This contains only the thoughts and sensations of which we are aware at any present moment. Next, there is the compartment known as "the preconscious." Here is stored every memory, every item of knowledge, that can be summoned to consciousness at will. Third, there is the compartment with which a psychiatrist tends to be especially concerned and which is usually called "the unconscious."

The contents of this compartment lie behind a barrier, the precise nature of which is not known. It may prove to be essentially chemical, electrical, or even purely psychological; but whatever its nature may prove to be, the effect is that material which lies behind the barrier can be brought across it into normal-waking-consciousness only with considerable difficulty.

Hypnosis is sometimes loosely spoken of as sleep, but this is inaccurate. Indeed, unless a specific suggestion is made to the contrary, a person under hypnosis may be unusually wide awake, in the sense that his powers of perception may be abnormally acute. But since such a person is not in a state of normal-waking-consciousness perhaps the best description of hypnosis is "a state of altered consciousness." An important feature of this state is that it weakens the barrier which confines the contents of the unconscious. This can be of particular value in psychiatry because it may enable the therapist to bring material from the patient's unconscious to the surface much more quickly than would otherwise be possible.

I have always considered myself fortunate in that at a very early stage I encountered a patient who illustrated the reality of the unconscious, and the power of material held in that compartment, in an unforgettable way.

The patient was a young woman who was wheeled into the ward in a chair because she had lost the use of her legs. A few days previously she had awakened in the morning to find that they were completely paralysed. Examination showed that there was nothing wrong with the nerves or muscles or bones, and that this was a paralysis of psychological origin.

In conversation she was clearheaded, calm, and indeed rather cheerful: surprisingly so for someone who, on the face of it, might never be able to use her legs again. We discussed many details of her life, including the fact that since her marriage she had become very disillusioned about her husband. However, for the previous year life had not been too bad because he had been abroad on business. Then, almost casually, she mentioned that a few days before the paralysis had occurred, she had received a letter which made her feel obliged to join him. She admitted that she was "a bit scared" at the prospect, but her principles demanded that nonetheless she should go. She added that her parents would be terribly distressed to learn that all was not well between her husband and herself.

Her voice had been level and matter-of-fact as she was telling me this. There was nothing to suggest a young woman striving to speak coherently while in a state of acute fear. But under hypnosis, when I brought the conversation round to her forthcoming trip, a very different picture emerged. She was not simply "a bit scared": she was terrified! And as details of the conditions she expected to find at the end of her journey also emerged, her fear was understandable. She was weeping and trembling, but through her sobs I heard her exclaim, "I would rather have no legs than have to go!"

I then brought her slowly back to normal-waking-consciousness, insisting as I did so that she remember all she had been telling me. Now that the full extent of her fear was in consciousness, she was scarcely recognizable as the poised young woman who had been wheeled into the ward. But now her problems were where we could explore them and cut them down to size.

We were able to discuss in exactly what respect her parents would be distressed to learn the true state of affairs, and it was not difficult to get her to consider rationally whether it was really necessary to stay with her husband. I was able to remind her that she had earned her living before her marriage and could easily do so again. By the end of this session she was very much calmer, and already had some power of movement in her legs.

During the next few days we had further talks along similar lines. Suddenly she declared that she had realised the significance of the paralysis of her legs. It was the only way in which she could avoid joining her husband without feeling that she was betraying what had been her principles. Within days after this session her legs were functioning perfectly normally.

I do not know if the wish to lose the use of her legs had ever been in her normal-waking-consciousness. But if it had been, and had remained entirely at that level, she would have been able only to fake a paralysis—a performance which she would have found impossible to sustain. But because it was flourishing in her unconscious, I was afforded a vivid demonstration of a principle which is often crucial in psychiatry: that an unconscious wish, if it is sufficiently powerful, may produce an effect that is tantamount to a physical fact. For her legs, temporarily, were as useless as if they had been amputated.

This case was instrumental in focussing my interest on an "analytically-orientated" approach to psychiatry. I use this rather cumbersome phrase because, while I acknowledge a debt to psychoanalytic theory, it contains certain cardinal principles which I have never been able to share. Therefore to describe my work as psychoanalysis would be inaccurate—and incidentally unjust, both to the psychoanalysts and to myself!

Very briefly, I accepted the concept that the memory of an event, which includes the sensations and emotions associated with it, might be stored in either the preconscious or the unconscious. If it were stored in the preconscious, from which it could readily be summoned to consciousness, then it became part of the total experience upon which the individual could base future decisions. The majority of our memories fall into this category; but those which are associated with so heavy a charge of unpleasant feelings that they would make life too uncomfortable if they were liable to recur unbidden to our awareness are relegated to the unconscious. Such feelings are not integrated; and instead of contributing to the source upon which we can draw at will, they have the power to force upon us the irrational ideas, feelings, and behaviour which comprise the symptoms which we call neurotic. One of the basic principles of therapy is to extricate these feelings and memories from the unconscious so that they can either be integrated or dissipated, and lose their power adversely to affect the personality. For this purpose I found the technique known as "hypnotic regression" particularly valuable.

To get a picture of what happens during regression

under hypnosis, consider the two ways in which a person in normal consciousness may speak of an incident which has happened to him. From his position in the present, he may simply be describing something which occurred in the past: in this case he will use the past tense, saying, "I was angry," "I was frightened," or "I was amused." But he may become so caught up in his story that he slips into the use of the present tense, and his gestures and the tone of his voice reveal that he is virtually reliving the episode. Either he has brought it up to the present or, and this may be the more apt explanation, he has temporarily left the present and merged himself with a past which for him is still extant.

Regression under hypnosis is an extension of this latter process. The subject may not only relive the incident as it occurred, but because of the breach which hypnosis may make in the barrier surrounding the unconscious, he may recover details of the event, and become aware of emotional facets, of which, on the original occasion, he was conscious only momentarily.

A vivid example of this mechanism was provided by a teen-age girl whose relationship with her parents was going through a very difficult phase. I had induced hypnosis for the first time during her therapy and simply to provide a starting point for the session, I asked her the name of her favourite tune. "I don't know any," she replied. This surprised me, because one of her mother's complaints had been that her daughter spent far too much money on gramophone discs.

I asked her how old she was. "I'm five," she said, and then burst into tears. She was already reliving an incident which had occurred when, at the age of five, she had fallen off a pony of which she was terrified. Her parents were urging her to remount; she was convinced that they were doing so only in the hope that she would fall off again and be killed!

The important feature of this regression was that although, in normal consciousness, she could have remembered falling from that pony, which she had distrusted and feared, the conviction that her parents wished her to die caused greater anxiety than she could tolerate, and this aspect of the incident, which was psychologically crucial, she had buried in her unconscious.

Such a spontaneous regression is rather unusual. Far more often, a regression is initiated by a specific suggestion from the therapist. I would tend to use this technique when a patient expresses feelings which seem grossly out of proportion to the event he is describing; for this is nearly always an indication that it has a significance for him in addition to its face-value. If the patient agrees that there is a question to be answered, I induce hypnosis and make a suggestion such as: "I am going to count slowly up to ten. While I am counting, you will go backwards in time, becoming younger and possibly smaller. When I reach ten, you will find yourself back in some situation which will help us to understand why the episode you have been describing meant so much to you."

On other occasions, having induced hypnosis, I would start the session by using one of the so-called "projection techniques." I would ask the patient to visualise a blank cinema-screen, and then tell him that, at the count of ten, a picture would appear on it which we would take as our starting point. When he had described the picture, I would use regression to help us to understand its relevance.

An apparently trivial episode may prove exceedingly useful. A girl of nineteen found herself back at the age of ten, playing Ping-Pong with her brother. I asked her the score. Without hesitation she replied, "Nineteen-seventeen." She was looking worried, so I asked what was the matter. She answered, "I think I am going to win, and he always gets so cross when I do."

Suddenly she brightened up. "Thank goodness! The dog has come in and we must stop playing because the cat is here already and they always fight." This small scene led us to her intense rivalry with her brother, which was an important factor in her illness.

The task of a therapist is to use his understanding of a particular case, his knowledge of psychological mechanisms, and his intuition, to judge whether an incident to which the patient has regressed is relevant or simply a cover story. In any event, the patient seldom reaches the crucial situation at the first attempt, and it is usually necessary, following approximately the same procedure, to induce him to go back still further.

I had become accustomed to seeing adult patients reliving events which had occurred when they were only three or four years old when a patient regressed to the age of two. She found herself being taken into her mother's bedroom to be introduced to her newborn brother. Fury was mounting within her at the sight of a baby nestling happily in the arms of *her* mother, when the nanny noticed a rash on her neck. The nanny, suspecting measles, whisked her back to the nursery. Measles it proved to be; in a sad little voice the patient declared, "I'm hot and sticky and red all over!" She interpreted her symptoms as the outward sign of the hostility she felt towards the new baby, and believed that she was being isolated as a punishment.

Shortly afterwards the same patient provided me with an experience which transcended anything I had previously encountered. The session had begun in a perfectly ordinary way. I had induced hypnosis, asked her to see a cinema screen, and on the screen to see a number. The number she saw was "5." I asked her if the number "five" meant anything to her. She thought for a moment and replied, "Only that I have five fingers."

"Anything special about your fingers?"

"Only that I bite my nails."

Nail-biting sometimes has a psychological significance and I felt that this might be a clue worth following up. So I told her that at the count of "twenty" she
would be back in a situation which would throw light
on her nail-biting. She found herself sitting in her
pram, aged nine months, wearing only a hat and biting
her thumb.

This regression was already to an earlier age than
had been reached by any of my patients, yet I felt sure
that there was still more to be uncovered. So I told her
that she would go further back, to a time when she was
biting something else.

Even as I was counting, she was becoming very red
in the face, pummelling the wall with her hands and
making violent sucking motions with her mouth. I
asked her to tell me what was happening.

"My mother is holding me to her breast to feed me,
but there is no milk coming out."

After some moments she gave a start of surprise.
Again I asked what was happening.

"She has put me over to the other side!"

The sucking and the pummelling of the wall were
resumed. Then there was another start of surprise,
followed this time by a wail and tears. "She's put me
down and gone away!"

A few days later, I had an opportunity of discussing
this session with the patient's mother. She declared at
once that the incident could very well have happened.
She had been unable to produce any milk, and in the
hope of stimulating a supply, had put the child to the
breast at each feed before giving her a bottle. But, on
the advice of her doctor, she had discontinued this
practice after three weeks. She was quite sure that she
had never spoken of this to her daughter; indeed the
whole matter had seemed so trivial that she doubted if
it had been mentioned to anyone.

She was entirely justified in considering it trivial:

41

innumerable infants must have had a similiar experience without any ill effects whatever. It had become significant only because of the way in which this patient had reacted to it.

This reaction was in fact quite complex. During the next two or three sessions I regressed her repeatedly to this incident, and it gradually became clear that although her mother had "put her down and gone away" only to fetch her bottle, the child had seen this in a completely different light. She had believed that her mother was deliberately withholding the milk, and that the anger she had felt on this account had caused her mother to vanish. Understandably, she developed a very exaggerated idea of the power of her anger; and this was a basic factor in her illness. As she gained this insight, her illness rapidly receded: and as she has not had a relapse in more than fifteen years to a condition which, with occasional intermissions, had crippled her life for the previous ten years, it seems justifiable to say that she was cured. It is pertinent, under the circumstances, to add that at the hospital where she had previously been treated, she had been advised that her only hope of relief lay in the operation of leucotomy.

I had never felt any doubt that this patient's regression to the age of three weeks had been genuine; and taking the other factors also into account, it seemed to me that I had irrefutable evidence, not merely that the mind was capable, at this early age, of registering and recording events, but that it was capable also of a complex reaction which might be the source of a neurosis in the future. To put the point the other way round, it seemed there was no doubt that a neurosis might result from the way in which an individual had reacted to an event when only three weeks old, and that through hypnotic regression it was possible to bring this event back to normal-waking-consciousness. With this in mind, during the next few months I caused a number of patients to regress to this early age,

42

and it became abundantly clear that their ability to do so was not even unusual.

The patient who took me the next step forwards—perhaps I should say backwards, was a woman of forty. She had been under treatment for several weeks when a session occurred in which she relived the experience of her birth. I had started the session by inducing hypnosis and asking her to see a picture. She saw the sand-dunes as they appeared from her bedroom window at home. As she uttered the words "sand-dunes," a strain of thought flashed through my mind: "Sand-dunes—shifting sands—here today and gone tomorrow—excellent symbol of insecurity—worth exploring." So I said to her, "At the count of 'ten' you will be back in a situation which has for you the same emotional significance of these sand dunes." I had no idea what her response might be, but when, on reaching "ten" I asked her where she was, she replied, "I am thirteen—at school. All the other girls are wearing summer frocks, but I am still wearing a winter one. I feel very embarrassed and out of place."

I asked her to go back further. "I am five. I am at a party and I want to go to the lavatory, but all the grown-ups are strangers and there is no one I can ask. I feel hot and uncomfortable." Still further back she finds herself in the basket of her brother's bicycle. He is taking her for a ride and swerving too fast round a corner. She feels very unsafe. At six months old she is in her pram, being taken for her first outing in the dark. The way lies through an avenue of pine trees which are swaying and creaking in the wind. She fears that one of the trees will fall on her and is very frightened. At the age of three weeks she finds herself in her mother's bed.

At this point came one of the small but intensely personal touches which, as one is observing a regression, give such a strong sense of validity. She is in her mother's bed because she has an earache. "My mother is putting her nipple in my ear to soothe it."

I asked her to go even further back to a time when she felt the same tone of emotion. She said, "I am very tiny. I seem to be lying on something very soft and white. I am very comfortable but somehow it is not right. I used to be part of a 'oneness' and now I am separated."

At this I told her that at "ten" she would find herself again part of the "oneness." As I reached "ten" she said, quietly and positively, "This is the womb." She went on: "There is something beating in me and through me—my mother's heart. I can't see—and it feels as if I have got no mouth." I asked her in what position she found herself. She replied "curled up," and immediately assumed the posture of a fœtus.

As she seemed perfectly comfortable, I left a nurse with her and went to fetch the medical superintendent to see this interesting phenomenon. While he watched, I told her that at the count of "ten" she would start to leave this place. At "ten" she arched her back, put one hand on her head, and an expression of severe suffering appeared on her features. She was portraying exactly what one can imagine a baby feels when the first contraction of the uterus clamps down upon it. In a moment or two this attitude was relaxed, only to be repeated some minutes later.

Her assumption of this attitude intrigued me. From time to time this patient suffered from a pain in her hip which was accompanied by a pain in her head, and had been subject to it for as long as she could remember. She had consulted numerous doctors, but none of them had been able either to account for or to relieve it. If an attack of the pain came while she was standing up, it would induce a particular gesture. She would put one hand on her head, the other on her hip and arch her back in a peculiar way. At the same time her face always assumed the same expression of acute distress. As nearly as her position curled up on the bed would permit, this was the posture and expression which she was now intermittently displaying.

Fearing that this stage might be as protracted as during the original confinement, I intervened and told her that she would move forward to actually leaving the womb. She began to moan from the pain in her head, and then, just as one felt that her head must soon emerge, she suddenly gasped, "I can't breathe!" and appeared to be fighting desperately for air. There came a short period of gasping and gulping, interspersed with cries that she could smell blood. It was exceedingly distressing to watch. Then, suddenly, she gave a great sigh of relief—"Ah...that's better!"—and appeared to fall asleep.

In due course I told her that I would count slowly to "twenty" and that as I was counting she would grow up to the present day. As I reached "five" she spontaneously uncoiled herself. I brought her out of hypnosis very gradually. Even so, she awoke with a blinding headache, which was only relieved by reinducing the state, suggesting very strongly that she would awaken without it, and then awakening her more slowly still.

In this particular instance, anybody who wished to do so could find theoretical grounds for protesting that there are other possible interpretations of this scene than a regression to the state of being unborn and the event of birth. For one thing, a close relative of the patient was a professional mid-wife. However, there is nothing to be gained by arguing the matter at this point, so I will merely reiterate my own belief that the regression was genuine.

On the basis of this belief, during the next two years I helped many patients to relive the experience of their birth. I became familiar with witnessing revivifications of such details as being born headfirst or tailfirst: of the head being gripped by forceps: of the patient being almost strangled by the cord being wound tightly round the neck. I think an unprejudiced observer would have considerable difficulty in explaining each one of these as either an "act" staged for my benefit, or the enactment, at my suggestion, not of a genuine experience of which the patient's mind had retained a record but of a fantasy based upon information they had acquired.

I also gained reason to believe that from at least as early as the fifth month of intra-uterine life the unborn baby is aware of itself as an individual. It is aware of its sex, of its position, of the length of time it has been in the womb, and of the relationship of its limbs to one another. One patient, who had had a most difficult birth, regressed to a period which he stated positively was the fifth month of intra-uterine life. He was aware that the cord had become wound round his neck, and also that his right arm had become trapped beneath his right leg. I have no obstetrical records to confirm this, but it would account most adequately for the difficulty experienced in delivering him.

I remained puzzled by the fact that patients often dated memorable intra-uterine events so positively until, ten years later, Joan offered what I think is the correct explanation: a mother is usually very conscious of the precise stage of her pregnancy, and the fœtus picks this up by telepathy.

By 1952, so many patients had relived details of their prenatal period that I no longer regarded it as anything remarkable. So when a patient who had been in therapy for several weeks told me she was sure that the cause of her illness lay in something which had happened before she was born, I replied that I would help her to find out what it was, not anticipating that anything out of the ordinary would come to light.

The patient was a young married woman in her mid-twenties. Her principal complaint was a depression from which she had been suffering for two years before she came into hospital. She had already revealed that one of her worst problems was a horror of anything to do with sex. Although she had two children, she had always been terrified of intercourse, and even had to leave a room if the conversation turned upon sexual matters.

She was an excellent hypnotic subject, and her fear of sex seemed a promising line along which to cause her to regress. She soon found herself back at the moment when she had just been born, and was choking from something wound tightly round her neck. She had no idea what this could be, and I asked her to trace it. Her hand went first to her neck, and then, as though running something between finger and thumb, it wandered down to her navel. "It comes from my tummy," she said.

A few moments later she exclaimed, "A man is injecting something into my arm!" She felt exceedingly frightened, and was quite sure that both the constriction round her neck and the injection were attempts on the part of her mother to get rid of her. When I had brought her out of hypnosis, she told me that even the idea of an injection had always filled her with acute alarm. It occurred to me that, in a symbolical sense, sexual intercourse fitted easily into this pattern.

At the next session, she declared that she would never get better until she discovered the origin of her feeling that her mother had not wanted her. Under hypnosis she affirmed that this had originated before she was born. This time, therefore, I regressed her straight back to the intra-uterine state. At once she appeared to be in great distress, moaning, "I'm burning! I'm burning!"

I asked her where she felt the pain. She replied, quite definitely, that it was in her stomach.

I told her that she would see something which would tell us how long she had been inside her mother. She saw first the word "seven," and then, in answer to my question "seven what?" she saw the word "months." She declared she was quite certain that the burning was caused by something which her mother was doing to try to get rid of her.

I then told her that if she had ever felt a similar sensation before, she would now go back to that earlier experience. I counted slowly to "ten," and again she moaned, "I'm burning! I'm burning!" This time she was equally definite that the pain was in her head.

I asked her how big she was. In a very faint voice she replied, "Very tiny...I cannot move my arms or my legs."

Again I asked her to see something which would tell us how long she had been in the womb. She saw the word "six," but this time, in response to my question, added the word "weeks."

Again she was certain that the burning was due to something her mother was doing in an attempt to get rid of her. At this point I told her that she would progress to the time of leaving her mother. As I was counting she suddenly appeared to be very worried. I asked her what was wrong, and she replied that she felt that there was something around her neck. She was able to pinpoint her intra-uterine age at five months.

As I reached "ten," she became very distressed indeed. She felt she was in a tunnel from which, despite frantic efforts, she was quite unable to escape. Then she felt someone get hold of her legs and pull them out. Next, something hard and painful grasped her head and began to twist it. Then, she was lying on something white and felt she was choking from something around her neck. She was aware of a man and woman, both dressed in white, and someone shrieking, "I don't want her! I don't want her!"

At this point I progressed her to the present day and brought her out of hypnosis. She recalled all that she had been through and insisted that it was as real to her as the memory of her breakfast. She knew very well what it was she had experienced, but she still had no idea what it was that had been around her neck. At the end of this session she looked, and felt, tired out.

To anticipate a little, this patient's mother, after the

end of the treatment, confirmed that her daughter had been born as a breech, and also that she had been nearly asphyxiated by the cord, which was wound tightly round the neck.

When the patient arrived for her next session, she greeted me with, "Do you know, Doctor, I feel somehow that it was my fault that my mother did not want me, but I must find out what it was that I did wrong."

I hypnotised her again, and began by putting to her once more the question, "Did this happen before or after you were born?" The answer was as positive as ever—"before." We had already been as far back as the sixth week of her pre-natal life and already, even at that early stage, she was quite certain that her mother did not want her. So I asked her, in a tone which I made as calm and level as I could, "Can you tell me whether this thing you did wrong occurred before you started to grow inside your mother or after? Was it after or before? Her reply was immediate, and again, very positive: "Before."

I asked her then, "Is it possible for you to recover this event?"

"Yes."

"How can I help you to recover it?"

"By counting to a hundred." So I counted quietly to a hundred, and asked her what she could tell me about herself. In a barely audible whisper she said, "I'm a tiny spot." She could tell me no more about herself than that, except that she was in a small place. Then she suddenly announced that she had moved to a larger place, and she knew that she had to touch something, "But it keeps moving away."

She repeated this phrase over and over again: "I should never have touched the thing that was moving!" After some minutes I interrupted and told her that I was going to bring her back to the present day: that I would count slowly from a hundred down to one, and that she would come forward in time to the present moment. From time to time I paused to ask her what was happening.

Immediately I started to count she began to grow bigger, though for a while she still remained "just a spot." Then she experienced once more the burning which had occurred at six weeks. At five months she again became aware that something was round her neck. I caused her to "leap-frog" over the experience of birth, and she found herself again on the white sheet, with the man and woman in white. From this point I brought her forwards fairly rapidly and out of hypnosis. She awoke utterly exhausted and looking completely bewildered. She said, "I know all that was real, but would you kindly tell me what it means?"

I had no doubt that she had been reliving her conception and her subsequent intra-uterine life. But I was reluctant to tell her this, and for the next half an hour or more I tried to lead her to realise this for herself by asking appropriate questions.

At this stage a most unexpected fact came to light. I was well aware that this patient had had only a very limited formal education which probably did not include any teaching of biology, but I was not prepared for her complete ignorance of the biological "facts of life." She was able to tell me that if you wanted a female rabbit to have young you would have to get a male rabbit too, but she had only the haziest idea of the role that each played in reproduction. She appeared to be completely ignorant of such things as spermatozoa and ova. Despite the fact that she had borne two children, she had no idea of the significance of the umbilical cord. To her, the navel was "something that happens when you are born."

This patient was of good average intelligence. I do not think that a wish to deceive me was a content of any part of her mind, conscious or unconscious. It is possible that when younger she had known all these things, but for some psychological reason had subsequently repressed the knowledge, but I do not think this is the case. I believe the explanation is that her fear of sex had been present from the very start of her life, and had had the effect of stifling all curiosity about anything connected with it. As she was under an anæsthetic when both her children were born, it is very probable that she had never seen an umbilical cord. It is just conceivable, though I did not ask about this, that she never saw either of her children naked until the stump of the cord had fallen off, in which case she could have remained ignorant of the significance of the navel.

Be that as it may, the most leading of questions failed to bring her nearer to any understanding, and eventually I offered to tell her what I believed she had been reliving.

Up to this time she had changed little from her condition prior to the start of treatment. She had seldom appeared severely depressed, but was completely listless. She would always do anything she was asked, but never showed any interest or enthusiasm for what she was doing. She seldom smiled, and her expression was always rather wooden. But as I began to tell her about the physiology of conception, a look of enlightenment started to dawn on her face which was profoundly moving. She had not the slightest doubt that her experience as "a tiny spot" was a reliving of the period before conception, and that "touching the thing that was moving" was the moment of conception itself. She exclaimed, "Now I understand what it was I did wrong! I was never meant to be born! That explains why I have never felt that there was a place for me in the world!"

She paused for a moment, looking thoughtful. But then, with a truly joyous note she went on: "But what does it matter that my mother never loved me! My husband does and so do my children! I have all the love any woman could want!"

On that note we ended the session. It had started at

eight in the evening and it was now close on midnight. Next morning she was still in bed. Understandably she looked very limp, but she was radiantly happy. The following morning, with a glint in her eye of which I would never have thought her capable, she said, "I want my husband!" He was in a different part of the country and could not reach her until the next day, when they went off together.

She called in to see me a week later. After eight years of marriage and two children they had been having their first real honeymoon, and she looked a different woman. Some weeks later she wrote to tell me that she had just had several teeth out under a local anæsthetic, and the injection had not worried her in the least.

Shortly after the patient had left the hospital her mother came to see me. As I have already recounted, she confirmed most of the details of the patient's birth as the patient had relived them. She denied ever trying to get rid of the child, but went on to tell me something which interested me far more than would have any admission of an attempt at abortion. Her husband's mother had been fanatically jealous of her, even before her marriage, and had threatened her with physical violence if she ever became pregnant. So her pregnancy had been a period of chronic fear, punctuated by more than one moment of panic when her mother-in-law had had to be physically restrained from trying to carry out her threats.

It seems to me entirely possible that the pain which the patient had felt when she "touched the thing that was moving" was in some obscure way related to the mother's dread of becoming pregnant. I feel sure that the episodes of "burning" which she had relived so vividly were the effects upon the unborn child of the moments of acute fear experienced by the mother. A physiological explanation of this might be that the mother's fear induced an outpouring of adrenaline into her bloodstream which then affected the fœtus.

But I did not need the corroboration of her mother's story to strengthen my conviction that the patient had relived her conception. The way in which the analysis had moved inexorably in this direction, added to the framework of my own understanding which had been extending steadily over the previous four years, left me in no doubt that this was what had happened.

I was exceedingly fortunate that this work took place with a patient whose personality was fundamentally very sound. I was also fortunate that the interval between the first occasion of encountering a regression to earlier than the fifth month of fœtal life and this patient's regression to her conception was very short. It was just possible to postulate that even at the fifth month the brain and nervous system were sufficiently developed to have carried out the mental activity of which I believed I had evidence: but a long drawn-out series of patients regressing successively to periods earlier than this would have been intellectually disquieting, for I was then still imbued with the idea that no part of an individual existed before his conception, and that there could not possibly be any form of mental function without a more or less fully developed brain. As it was, I was confronted with a series of regressions which bridged the period from birth to conception in three sessions. Clinically and intuitively I had accepted their validity, which was surely justified by the results: but before I had had time to speculate upon how they could have been possible the answer had arrived in my head: in a human being there must be an element which exists and is capable of function even in the absence of a physical body!

The concept of such a non-physical component, under one name or another, must be as old as mankind, but it was tremendously exciting to have reached it for myself through a series of experiences which had been acceptable to my intellect. I felt as though I had arrived at a clearing in a forest from which paths could be seen to run in a variety of directions, promising to lead towards the answers to such questions as the relationship of Mind to Body, the nature of Memory, and so on. But, not surprisingly, a new question now presented itself: "What is the origin of this component?"

It might be imagined that reincarnation dropped neatly into place as an entirely acceptable answer, but in fact this was not the case. There were, I think, several reasons. Probably the most telling was my assumption that since the body was initiated by a contribution from each parent, the psyche, as I then called the non-physical component, would be formed in a similar way. This error caused me to misinterpret my patient's reliving of her conception, to the extent that I assumed she was reliving the meeting of the sperm and the ovum, instead of, as I now believe was the case, the moment when her personality contacted the fertilised egg. I had, in fact, a mental picture of "half-psyches" bestriding the germ-cells like jockeys! However, artificial insemination made this difficult to sustain. I could not imagine several million "half-psyches," each perched precariously on a sperm, waiting in a bottle in a refrigerator until some operator gave them the "Off!"

On the other hand, I could not see a really acceptable alternative. It was undeniable that children inherited physical characteristics from their parents, and I still assumed, mistakenly, that certain traits of personality for which the body could not be held responsible were also inherited. The idea of a long personal history was obscured from me by Jung's concept of the "Universal-unconscious," which seemed so adequately to explain such phenomena as a man who had lived all his life in the depths of the country dreaming about the sea.

During the next six years, I encountered patients whose anxiety I still found myself unable to explain even after the most exhaustive scrutiny of their life-story in terms of classical psychoanalytic theory. Such cases caused me to wonder whether it was possible for an individual to inherit anxiety from a parent, but it still did not cause me to think in terms of earlier lifetimes of his own. Thus although my thoughts returned time and again to the question of where the psyche had come from, the rigidity of my own thinking prevented me from making any satisfactory progress.

Then, one evening early in 1958, I was talking with a chance acquaintance, an aeronautical scientist, about extra-sensory perception. I described to him an occasion when a patient who was deeply under hypnosis had apparently been able to project her mind to my home and to describe certain features of it with remarkable accuracy.

Her first comment had been that there seemed to be a double hedge round it. In fact, the garden was enclosed by a hedge, inside which was a fence I had erected because the hedge was not thick enough to contain my boxer bitch.

She then said, "There is a lawn in front of the house and there are several small trees on it." This was accurate; I had recently planted some apple trees on this lawn, which was about the size of a lawn-tennis court.

Her next remark was surprising. "It is dark, and I cannot find my way into the house." I had overlooked the fact that this session was taking place late on a winter evening. Furthermore, the front door was recessed and set at an unusual angle. Several visitors had found it difficult to locate at night if the light above it had not been switched on.

I had been impressed by this small experiment. But my acquaintance accepted it calmly, merely observing that he believed there had been eras when a great deal more had been known about such forms of perception than was the case today. He went on to tell me that the faculty my patient had displayed had been used in early dynastic Egypt as we now use radar. He then asked me if I had read any books by Joan Grant.

I replied that I had never heard of them, whereupon he told me that this author had the faculty of being able to recall many of her earlier lives, and that seven of her books were, in fact, posthumous autobiographies. Such a faculty was far beyond the point to which my own work had brought me, but I felt a sense of great excitement; a sense that a door was about to open upon far more than merely the answer to a philosophical problem.

Before I had finished *Winged Pharaoh,* the book I read first, I knew, beyond any possibility of doubt, that reincarnation was a reality. It would be futile to try to account for this feeling of certainty in terms of pure reason. Only later did intellect bridge the gap between my own researches and an intuitive conviction that I had been reminded of a fundamental pattern of evolution which I had long known to be true.

I would have journeyed halfway round the world to meet the author, but fortunately such a long pilgrimage proved unnecessary. I soon learned that Joan was living only thirty miles away. I met her on the 14th of May. I came to dinner and left at three o'clock in the morning. Seldom can so many words have been exchanged in eight hours.

As I had anticipated, my experience with hypnosis linked with Joan's knowledge and experience of reincarnation as effortlessly as a river meets the sea. But as the autobiography of her present life covers only the period up to 1937, I did not know that during the war years she had worked closely with a psychiatrist and had acquired considerable psychiatric experience. This was an entirely unexpected bonus.

It seemed to be absurd that the fullest possible use should not be made of her faculties, while she wished for nothing more than the opportunity to resume regular work in this field. So, before I left, we had already discussed tentative plans for working together. We neither of us foresaw that within two months we should have embarked upon life together also.

3

THE SUPRA-PHYSICAL BODY

by Joan Grant

Implicit in the recognition of reincarnation is the knowledge that the current personality is not only immortal, but is one of a series of personalities. But it is less generally recognized that the body, except for its outer, three-dimensional rind, is equally immortal.

The body of every individual has a physical and a supra-physical component; and when the energy exchange between these two components ceases to exist, the physical body dies. But the supra-physical body does not die. It cannot die: for the simple reason that it consists of an order of matter which is not subject to the process which we call "death," a process during which the physical particles integrated by an energy field disintegrate because the energy field has become inactive.

The majority of misconceptions about the conditions of discarnate life have stemmed from the illusion that the only aspects of the personality which can exist independently of the physical body are those concerned with concepts and emotions. If this were so, the dead would indeed be amorphous, creatures without passion or parts; but fortunately such apparitions exist only in the imagination, or in Gothic tales.

The true state of affairs is that the supra-physical

body is the receptor of sensory experience on all its levels of activity, and when free of the need to operate through its physical counterpart is infinitely more perceptive than when muffled in flesh. So the personality, whether the physical body happens to be dead or alive, awake or asleep, conscious or unconscious, always retains both form and function.

The knowledge that we have "bodies terrestrial and bodies celestial" is by no means new. It was a commonplace in more enlightened civilizations such as early dynastic Egypt, which is why the Sphinx, the body of an animal with a human head, symbolizing the dual aspects of the personality, was so often depicted in the Nile Valley.

It is because dogmatists, who could not accept a nonmaterial reality, confused the supra-physical with the physical body, that the concept of the resurrection of the material particles came to be grafted onto the Christian heritage.

The same disastrous misbelief has caused death to assume a grotesque stature in our modern civilization. Morticians may benefit from the prevalence of necrophobia, but hundreds of thousands of individuals suffer exceedingly because their physical bodies are kept ticking over, by chemical and sometimes even by mechanical means, when they are obviously ready to be shed, just as a snake sheds its outgrown skin.

As though it were not bad enough to deny immortality to the more subtle aspects of the body, a further indignity was added—the body was portrayed not as the essential partner but as the enemy of other elements of the personality. Vast numbers of people, although paying lip-service to a divine creation, were duped into denying and otherwise persecuting their bodies. This is a particularly malign practice, since the body which has become habituated to inflicting suffering on itself is unlikely to be squeamish about inflicting suffering on the bodies of others.

Unfortunately this malign practice is still considered respectable by many otherwise sane members of society. Ritual flagellation or hair shirts are now unusual means of auto-torture, but those addicted to the same unhealthy attitude of "strength-through-suffering" can expect to be seen as heroic by the majority of their audience.

To deny, instead of striving to develop, any of our five senses, instead of training them to be instruments through which to give and receive joy, is as misguided as would be the musician who thought he would play the piano better if he cut off one of his hands. But a pernicious process of conditioning has caused many people to feel admiration for anyone who is making himself deliberately uncomfortable. The boxer, for instance, who takes punishment until he is concussed once too often and becomes half-witted; the climber who climbs on although he risks losing fingers and toes through frostbite; the fakir on his bed of nails and the celibate in his cell. Why is there such a strong tendency to see their self-inflicted miseries as an indication of merit?

The reason is simple, but not particularly flattering. It is because nearly everybody, at one time or another, has indulged in such futile misuse of energy. So it requires considerable, and often very humbling, reassessment of our ideas, and a courageous mobilization of our innate honesty, before we realize, once and for all, that there is no virtue whatsoever in seeking suffering.

I have learned this by personal experience. For instance there was an occasion when I was so careless of my body's survival that I insisted on voicing my beliefs, although I knew that by so doing I would make no dent in the wall of dogma by which the people of that century had allowed themselves to be imprisoned. So I was burned alive: which is an exceedingly unpleasant way of being murdered. But at least no one else suffered; and the crowd found a witch-burning as stimulating as a contemporary crowd finds a crash in an automobile race.

However, I was not always lucky enough only to damage myself. In the twelfth century, I caused a handsome and healthy body of which I was fond to inflict gross discomfort on itself and others by donning armor and jousting with similarly deluded males. Eventually that body died by having a poignard driven through its right eye...an episode I still remember too vividly for comfort.

I think what keeps the memory so clearly defined is the shocked amazement I felt when my visor was opened, and instead of seeing the smiling face of my squire, about to unbuckle my harness and help me to my feet, I saw the face of my vanquished opponent's squire, who in a moment of vengeful anguish proceeded to dispatch me. I felt even sorrier for myself shortly afterward. For instead of being praised for my devotion to the laws of chivalry, I was told, very briskly indeed, that I would have lived far closer to the benign pattern of evolution if I had listened to the advice of my sensory experience...which had implored me to stay at home, to cultivate my garden and the love of my wife.

Even among people who are fully aware that their current personality is only one of a long series it is not unusual to find that they regard their earlier bodies as castoff clothes, worn for a life-span and then discarded. When asked to explain why some bodies are born with inherent health and beauty, and others are crippled, a frequent answer is to the effect that the body is given to us either as a reward or as a punishment. But our body is not given to us: it is initiated by an earlier superphysical of our own, although not necessarily its immediate forerunner in the series.

The raw material which a superphysical affects when organizing a new physical body is a fertilized ovum and its genes. A fertilized ovum has its own energy, but only sufficient to keep it alive for two or three days, unless it is adopted by a superphysical. If the super-physical has taken on this particular ovum after due forethought and by deliberate choice, it can make an efficient selection from the available genes. It is in fact choice not chance which has made a particular child far healthier and better looking than other siblings of the same family.

The alert superphysical will also influence the mother so that she instinctively desires the type of food the growing embryo needs. If the embryo is being dis-tressed by her over-smoking or too many martinis, the supra-physical will probably afflict her with a distaste for them, and if this fails to abate the nuisance, may resort to giving her bouts of nausea until she takes the hint. But if the supra-physical grabbed the first fertil-ized ovum it could find, so as to scuttle back to a physical environment, it will probably make such an inept selection from the available material that the body which results will be far less admirable than it might have been.

It is the Integral, the sum-total of the wisdom ac-quired through the whole series of personalities, who should decide which supra-physical should organize the new body which will become the physical compo-nent of the incarnating personality. There will be an instinctive resonance between the supra-physical which has acted as a "parent" to the fœtus and the incarnating individual: which is why the physical skills acquired in one particular preexistence are usu-ally more easily available than the skills acquired in any of the others.

The supra-physical which has been selected by the Integral will nearly always organize a fœtus of its own sex. But if a supra-physical which has become split off from its Integral impulsively attaches itself to a fertil-ized ovum it may create a fœtus of the opposite sex with only partial success; which is the cause of certain types of sexual anomaly. For instance, a woman who has suffered many unwanted pregnancies, or who has died in terror after an abortion or childbirth, may protect herself from a repetition of such an agonizing experience in several different ways. She may make her new body infertile; or, if she decides to become male, may make it either impotent or sterile, so that she will not be able to inflict similar miseries on anyone else. She may decide to be immune to sexual desires except with a member of the same sex, whether this be male or female. This is a very common cause of homosexuality, and if it were generally recognized not only would cure be facilitated but the infliction of further unhappiness by ignorant critics would be avoided.

Although the physical body can be affected by innumerable outside causes, such as being cured of sepsis by an antibiotic, or paralysed by the virus of poliomyelitis, the supra-physical is very seldom affected except by causes within the personality. Therefore a man deafened by bomb-blast would retain his hearing on all other levels of reality. But a man who became deaf rather than hear the nagging voice of his wife might find the perception of his supra-physical ears also diminished. And he may remain under this self-imposed disability until he recognizes that instead of resorting to the craven device of making himself deaf he should have caused his wife to stop bullying him or else left her.

A frequent cause of damage to the supra-physical body is a concept held by another component of the personality. For instance, if the body, guided by its innate wisdom, finds another body repellent, yet is forced to endure intimate contact because its instincts have been overruled by the false ethics held by the rest of the personality, trouble will inevitably ensue. This may appear as mental or as physical disease, neither of which is likely to be relieved until the individual has changed his concept of "duty."

Duty, which is so often the excuse for doing something we know to be wrong, causes an appalling number of people to endure intercourse as a drab routine, simply because they are labelled "wife" and "husband." They are thereby inadvertently committing "adultery," for the original meaning of this term was "sex without joy"—an illuminating fact told to me by one of the few real priests I have met in this century, who was also a renowned biblical scholar. He died shortly before he was to have been ordained as a bishop of the Church of England, and used to thunder from the pulpit, "Ninety-nine percent of adultery takes place in the marriage-bed!"

If a celibate prays with sufficient fervor for the "gift of continence" he may render his supra-physical impotent. Unless he realized his error before he died, or during his excarnate period asks to be relieved of his disability, it is probable that a later body will suffer from this malfunction. Unfortunately, people who have prayed for something which they later realize to be the last thing they really wanted, often find that false pride prevents them from asking to be cured. However well intentioned and efficient a healer may be, and whatever the level of consciousness on which he is operating, cure cannot take place without the cooperation of the patient. Eventually even the most stubborn will become sufficiently distressed to ask for help, even though this may entail having frankly to admit that only blind obedience to dogma or terror of taboo caused them to waste a great deal of time and energy on their knees.

Many apparently irrational fears have their origin in some painful episode experienced by an earlier supra-physical which the current body is determined not to repeat. A trivial instance of this mechanism caused me to be unable to learn to dive. In spite of a passionate determination to overcome the disability which forced me to walk furtively down the steps of a swimming-bath while other young women poised elegantly on the diving board, I invariably jerked my head back before it touched the water. I did innumerable belly-flops before I finally had to accept that I did not know how to stop my body resonating to an earlier one, who had accidently broken his neck on a submerged rock.

A few years ago I tried to cure my terror of snakes by getting Charles to catch a slow-worm so that I could accustom myself to handling it. Having organized this experiment I was confident that I could carry it through, especially as I knew the reptile was entirely harmless. I was not conscious of any anxiety, in fact I was mildly embarrassed that I had decided to practice on a slow-worm instead of starting with a proper snake.

I can recall the incident so vividly that I can almost see my hand as it stretches out to pick up the little slow-worm, curled so confidingly on Charles' palm. Then my hand stops in midair, the fingers spread out as though pressing against a pane of glass. I spent nearly an hour trying to touch that slow-worm; feeling more and more foolish and becoming increasingly angry with myself. But I could not force my hand within six inches of it. My intellect knew that I was in no danger: but my body, reso-nating to experience stored in earlier supra-physicals, knew that agonizing pain resulted from snakebite.

I am sure that the fear of snakes is so commonplace only because the majority of us have had distressing encounters with their widespread species during our long-history. But as I then believed that bringing any type of unpleasant memory into normal-waking-conscious-ness would defuse its latent energy, I embarked on the recall of three snakebite episodes, two of which had resulted in premature death. Had these episodes resulted in fragment of the personality becoming split off, the recall would almost certainly have had a therapeutic effect. However, as they had long since been integrated, bringing then into my field of awareness temporarily made matters worse and I gained nothing from this effort except yet another example of the occupational risks of far-memory.

Experience stored in many supra-physicals not only warns the current body against repeating an action which has proved disastrous but also tries to protect it from suffering through demands made upon it by the intellect. For instance, if my body is becoming stiff because I have been crouching too long over a typewriter, it would, if given half a chance, instinctively stand up and stretch. But too often my intellect, engrossed in trying to express an idea, refuses to take notice of my body's sensible suggestion which has been politely put forward as a whisper of mild discomfort. If this request continues to be ignored, the body will announce its need more vehemently as pain. This is why it is important to be aware of one's body instead of studiously ignoring its advice: a subject which is discussed in greater detail in the chapter on the cultivation of instinct.

The recognition that pain is primarily a warning, and an appeal for help, being transmitted by the supra-physical body to other components of the personality, can have practical applications in various forms of pain-reducing techniques. One of these techniques I began to use in my early twenties, although at the time I had not worked out the rationale of the process and was acting only instinctively.

An acquaintance told me that she was to undergo major abdominal surgery for the removal of a massive growth which was thought to be malignant. She wanted me to be with her before she went to the operating theatre and when she came round from the anæsthetic, because she felt that I could be trusted to tell her whether she had a chance of making a good recovery, or whether she should relinquish her body as smoothly as possible. She was afraid of going under anæsthetics, which she took badly, and had previously suffered prolonged vomiting which caused her wound to burst after a simple appendectomy.

I was with her when the nurse gave her Avertin and she drifted into unconsciousness as though into a natural sleep, a perfectly normal occurrence. The operation took over two hours and the outcome was far better than any of us had expected: for the growth was a fibroid weighing nearly four pounds but free from any trace of malignancy.

When she was brought back to her private ward, in which I was waiting, she was, of course, still deeply unconscious: and the nurse urged me to go out to lunch as the patient would not come round for three or four hours. I was about to do so, when I had a hunch that I should stay with her and that no one else should be in the room. Before I could achieve this privacy, I had to get both the surgeon and the physician to tell the matron that I did so with their full approval.

Again acting on hunch rather than by logic, I drew a chair to the bedside so that I could sit comfortably relaxed with my hand on her forehead. Then I proceeded to tell her, speaking slowly and clearly, exactly what had been done to her body...the surgeon had been kind enough to tell me the procedure he had followed in considerable detail. I knew that she was oblivious to the sound of my voice, but the words acted as a carrier-wave which made it easier to impress her supra-physical with the information I was striving to convey.

Having emphasized that she need no longer have any fear of cancer, I described the muscle layers which had been divided, and the various other tissues which had been cut and then sutured during the course of the operation so that she knew exactly where to direct the energy which would accelerate their healing. I explained that the warning sent to her consciousness in the form of pain had been acted upon, and that therefore the pain was no longer useful. I then told her that instead of seeing the anæsthetic as an enemy which had driven her out of her body, she would accept it as the benign agent which had prevented her from feeling the pain of surgery. Therefore instead of trying to get rid of its residues by vomiting, she would use them as an anodyne which would cause her to prolong her anæsthesia into a state of natural sleep.

Every few minutes I repeated the performance: which further experience with other postoperative patients has proved to be unnecessary unless the patient is particularly unreceptive.

For a period of four hours she hardly stirred: in itself an excellent sign, for before the development of modern improvements in anæsthesia, an unconscious patient often threshed about, thereby putting a strain on the stitches, and sometimes had to be restrained from falling out of bed. She awoke only long enough to say drowsily, "It was so silly of me to imagine it might be cancer....I don't in the least want to throw up...so I'll go back to sleep."

She slept peacefully all through the night: and even on the first postoperative day suffered such minor discomfort that this was easily controlled with aspirin instead of morphia. Her wound healed so rapidly that she was convalescing in my London house within a week.

An example of a different technique by which energy directed at a supra-physical can affect the physical body was provided by a man of twenty-three who came to Trelydan. I had advertised for a tutor, and among the replies was a letter from the almoner of the plastic surgery unit at East Grinstead, saying that they had a patient who had already undergone several operations but was still suffering from osteomyelitis of the right shinbone which would eventually require the amputation of his foot. However, before this could be done satisfactorily it was considered advisable that he should have at least three months' holiday in which to regain his strength, and that he would benefit from a peaceful environment where he could have good food and fresh air. He would need minimal nursing care: his dressing would have to be changed by a medical practitioner every second day, but this could be done in the doctor's surgery.

His medical papers were sent to our local doctor, who told me that it would be useless to try to do more for the boy than to feed him well and keep him cheerful: for in those days, before penicillin, osteomyelitis was an intractable condition. The day after the boy arrived I took him down to the evening surgery, intending to watch the wound dressed so that I could learn how to do it for him myself. However the sight and stench of yards of pus-soaked packing being pulled from a four-inch cavity in the bone made me feel so faint that I only just managed to get out of the room without either doctor or patient realizing my inadequacy.

The boy was tired when we got home and decided to have dinner in bed. He gladly accepted my suggestion that I should assist him to get in and out of his bath, and recounted the history of each of his many scars which he regarded quite objectively as a kind of battle diary. He had received them all on the first day of active combat and had lain all night in the desert before being picked up. He had been hit by seven different bullets. One had nicked a kidney, another a lung, two more had gone through his shoulder blade; and the other three had been relatively superficial, including the one which had chipped his shinbone just above the ankle. From all the major and two of the minor wounds he had made a surprisingly rapid recovery and suffered very little sepsis. But the shin had become seriously infected and had already extended his period in hospital by several months.

Having taken down his dinner tray and seen him settled with a book, I joined Charles and Bill Kennedy, a close friend of Jung, in my study, where they had retreated from the rest of the house-party to enjoy the last bottle of really good port. I cannot now remember what we were talking about, except that it was not concerned with the boy or his leg, when I suddenly exclaimed, "Don't talk for a minute....I have shifted level."

I found myself looking at a more than life-size crucifix, carved in wood and vividly colored, the wounds as though dripping with fresh blood. Kneeling in front of it, his eyes fixed on the nail driven through the feet, was a young monk who I knew to be a previous personality of the boy who was reading in the bedroom upstairs. I knew that the young monk was praying to receive a sign of grace in the form of stigmata: but being afraid of seeming lacking in humility he asked that this sign should appear not on his hands or his forehead but on his feet.

My level-shift lasted only for a couple of minutes, but as I returned to normal consciousness I realized that the wound in the boy's ankle had coincided exactly with the nail driven through the outer foot of the figure on that agonizingly realistic crucifix. I was vague about the date and the other circumstances; but thought the monk was Spanish and that he had died unshriven, probably while on a mission to South America in the eighteenth century.

I knew, with that inner certainty which is much more valid than logic, that the monk's supra-physical would release its energy, and therefore its capacity to affect the boy's body, only by being given the symbol of absolution which he would recognize. He required the freedom conferred by a properly charged eucharist. So taking a glass of port and a biscuit I held my hands over them and prayed very intently that I might be the vehicle of the necessary blessing.

I had already discovered that the boy had no interest whatever in reincarnation or in any allied subject. He had been brought up in a very puritanical family, which had caused him to dislike any form of religion;

and he had been obviously relieved to learn that none of us went to church. So I took him what purported to be an entirely mundane glass of port and a biscuit.

Forty-eight hours later I again took him to have his dressing changed. The doctor told me afterwards that he could hardly believe his eyes or his nose when he drew from the wound perfectly clean, dry packing; and saw that in the depths of it there was already healthy granulation. There was no recurrence of sepsis nor did the boy suffer any further pain in his leg. However the damage to the bone was so extensive that it remained too fragile to bear his weight evenly; and two years later he decided that he would walk better with an artificial foot. So he had it amputated, and from this operation he made an uneventful recovery.

Another case in which an earlier supra-physical was being troublesome concerned a psychiatrist, Alec Kerr-Clarkson. He first came to Trelydan because he had a tentative interest in the possibility of reincarnation through material he had collected from his patients undergoing hypnoanalysis. Subsequently he had read two or three of my books and thought I might be an interesting subject for further research.

He was on the point of leaving the house to catch a night train back to the north of England, after a mutually enjoyable but uneventful weekend, when Charles gave him a brace of pheasants. As rationing was then at its most strident, pheasants were usually a most welcome gift, so we were both surprised when instead of taking the birds, which were tied together by the neck with a loop of string, Alec looked very embarrassed and backing away asked that the birds should be wrapped securely in a parcel. Charles, mystified, explained that the birds would travel better unwrapped; at which Alec exclaimed, "But I can't touch feathers!"

The words were hardly out of his mouth before I heard myself saying emphatically, "The reason you can't touch feathers is because you had a death which was very similar to one of mine. You were left among the dead on a battlefield....I don't know where or when...but the ground was arid, pale sand and outcrops of grey rock. Vultures are watching you...six vultures. You are very badly wounded, but you can still move your arms. Every time you move, the vultures hop a little further away. But then they hop closer again....Now they are so close that you can smell them...they are beginning to tear at your flesh...."

At this point Charles interrupted me; for Alec was clearly distressed. He had collapsed onto the sofa and was sweating profusely. He was obviously in no condition to travel and thankfully accepted our suggestion that he remain at least until the following day. He went up to his room, but soon called me.

Although he had tried to stop his violent shivering by having a hot bath, and had put himself to bed, he was still in the grip of a spontaneous recall. He exhorted me to drive the vultures away, and waved his arm as though he could still see them hopping inexorably towards him...."Why did they leave me to die alone...why?...why? Every other man had a friend to cut his throat...why did they betray me....Me!" His terror had been replaced by a rising fury of indignation.

Suddenly I realized that it was this emotion which had caused him to become bound to his death by vultures. He felt that he had suffered not just a horrific death, but the betrayal by his comrades, who had left him to die alone on the battle field. I should have realized this sooner, for I knew only too well that it was the duty of a man-at-arms' immediate superior to kill those who were seriously wounded rather than to leave them to die slowly...such a *coup de grace* even conferred a form of shriving if there were no priest available to give absolution.

I spent most of this night sitting on his bed, while he alternately shivered and sweated as though suffering from a bout of malaria. But at last I was able to make the man he had been realise that he had not been deliberately abandoned, and he said with infinite relief, "They must have thought I was dead....I am not angry any more....I have no reason to hate them for leaving me to die among the dead...." Then he was Alec and no one else, and he went quietly to sleep.

He slept until noon, to wake refreshed and free from symptoms. Not until later that day did he tell me that he had had a phobia about feathers since childhood. He had found this so embarrassing, especially as his children teased him for not even being able to rescue birds which had got caught in the strawberry nets, that he had sought help from several colleagues, who were as ineffective in curing him as he had been in his efforts to cure himself. When he left to catch the night train he was carrying the pheasants by their necks. In his bread-and-butter letter he wrote, "I hope none of my fellow passengers knew I was a psychiatrist because they would have thought my behavior very odd for a member of my profession. I could not resist the temptation of taking the pheasants down from the rack and stroking them...for I was so delighted to show myself that I now actually enjoy touching feathers!"

Although the physical body has no reality except in the immediate present, for today's version has replaced yesterday's, which has therefore ceased to exist, this law does not apply to earlier versions of its supra-physical component. For these supra-physical components, being immune to the process of death, can maintain an independent identity so long as the personality provides them with sufficient energy to do so. In practice it is unusual to find an individual in whom several supra-physicals do not coexist.

Multiple supra-physicals can be a valuable asset to the personality, providing it not only with a wider field of activity, but also facilitating identification with people of different age groups. They allow the personality not only to remember, but actually to experience the sensory awareness which their physical body registered only at an earlier phase of its existence. Using the supra-physical which developed when one was a child is by far the best way of communicating with children: for except in the strictly three-dimensional sense, one is again feeling as a child feels, and not as a grown-up. A wider application of the same mechanism is also to use the supra-physicals belonging to earlier personalities. This makes it much easier to identify with people older than oneself, or who are of a race to which one no longer belongs; or the opposite sex.

If these supra-physicals, when not in use, contain only the energy required to maintain their identity, they are comparable to a wardrobe full of clothes which are available for any appropriate occasion. But if any of them contains an undue amount of energy, which it cannot, or will not, release, this energy can cause trouble to the rest of the current personality; or to a later one in the same series.

If the body of an adult is receiving its movement orders from a supra-physical created during childhood, the discrepancy in the relative size of these two components may render the individual accident prone. Instead of moving smoothly together, like a well-matched pair of trotting horses, they are as uneasy as a Percheron in double harness with a Shetland pony.

I had recognized this intuitively on several occasions, years before the concept of the supra-physical body had taken shape, and therapy based on this intuition had been successful. The first time I used it was with a boy of sixteen who was pathologically clumsy. When he climbed trees he usually misjudged the distance between one branch and another, or relied on one too fragile to bear his weight. He fell off his bicycle, bumped into furniture, stumbled downstairs, and the crash of breaking plates was a sure sign the he was helping to wash the dishes.

I was bringing him home from the doctor's surgery, where he had endured having six stitches put into a cut knee with his usual stoicism, when I had a sudden hunch about the cause of his trouble. While their children were small, his parents were demonstratively affectionate: but the moment they were old enough to go to boarding school, at seven, then they were expected to be manly. In their terms "manly" meant not only being physically tough, but foregoing the warm physical contact which is such a vital factor in expressing and receiving affection.

After dinner that evening he was lying on the sofa in my study, and under the guise of seeking his advice, I embarked on the case history of an imaginary colonel. The colonel's symptoms were seen to be the result of his following the stiff-upper-lip tradition which had led to his being incapable of expressing his feelings. By the time I had finished, there was little left of this heroic figure except the medal ribbons on his battle-dress. He was shown to be less of a man than a marionette, and he appeared brave only because his imagination had become so parched that he could not believe a bullet would hit him. As the boy was in the throes of his first love affair, I provided the colonel with a wife, who had confided to me that her husband was not only a ghastly bore in public but even more boring in bed.

As I finished, the boy suddenly flung his arms round me and sobbed. But his tears were tears of relief—at realizing that there was nothing in the least juvenile in being lovable and longing to be loved.

His clumsiness had been due to his trying to perpetuate the period of his life in which it had been respectable to be hugged. The moment he recognized that to appear unfeeling was not only misguided but frankly unhealthy, his energy was freed to flow into his

75

current supra-physical, with the result that his coordination improved with astonishing rapidity. He proved this the following morning by washing a collection of fragile antique glass without chipping any of it: and the next term at school he revealed an unexpected aptitude for cricket and squash rackets. But what pleased him far more was that he found he could dance very well, instead of alienating his girl friends by trampling on their feet.

A similar mechanism was at work in another patient. He was exceptionally tall, but despite the fact that he had several times hit his head on low doorways, and even when getting into his own automobile, hard enough to cause severe concussion, at least one painful bang on the forehead was a daily occurrence.

I applied salves and sympathy, until he suddenly received from me a more brusque form of therapy... which does me no credit as it was inspired by sheer exasperation. He had offered to take up a child's supper tray, and a couple of minutes later I heard a crash followed by an ominous thud which sent me running upstairs. He had hit his head on the low beam and knocked himself out. I thought at first that he had split his skull, for his head looked a gory mass which only on further investigation proved to be mainly tomato soup.

As I was the only other adult in the house, I dragged him inch by inch along the corridor and heaved him onto his bed. He remained unconscious while I pulled shards of pottery out of his face, applied sticking-plaster and generally cleaned him up. At this point he opened his eyes and said fretfully, "I wish you'd had the sense not to live in a house designed for midgets."

I had heard variations of this complaint once too often. "It wasn't designed for giants who pretend to be midgets!" I retorted. "How many more times must you make a nuisance of yourself, before you accept the fact that you are six foot six, not five foot high!"

"I am *not* tall!" he said indignantly. Then he added

more slowly, "At least I don't feel tall...I suppose I feel about the size I used to be when I was a boy of fourteen."

It took two or three weeks to unravel why his body image had stuck at this period of his life, but when we had done so he felt his true size and so ducked automatically.

Although a "stuck" or outgrown supra-physical can make a nuisance of itself, one which is free and efficient can provide, among other advantages, a most useful means of teaching a skill to the physical component. This I discovered when, at the age of sixteen, I broke the tendons which support the arch of my left foot. The prognosis was gloomy, and I was depressed by having overheard a doctor tell my mother that I should never be able to dance again or play tennis, although I might eventually walk well enough to play golf.

This seemed very cold comfort, as I had shown such minimal aptitude after half-a-dozen lessons that the golf pro had stated that it would be a waste of his time and Father's money to give me any further instruction.

After some sixteen weeks of lying on sofas or being pushed round the garden in an ancient Bath chair, with the added misery of being unable to play the piano as I had developed a temporary paralysis in my arms through using crutches, I decided that I would try to teach myself to play golf by practicing it in my supra-physical—which in those days I thought of as my "upstairs body." With the patience of a performing seal learning to balance a ball on its nose I taught each muscle to play its part in the act. Over and over again I imagined myself playing round the links, which I could visualize as I had often walked round with those of my young men who were keen golfers. For two months, both when awake and asleep, I practised golf assiduously. I now only had to prove that I could repeat the performance on the three-dimensional level of activity.

Fortunately the Hampshire County Championship was played at Hayling Island that year. The plaster was taken off my foot four days before the meeting. I got a friend to enter my name for each event, and obtained Mother's permission to go to the clubhouse, on the excuse that I wanted to watch the players driving off.

When I advanced onto the first tee, part of my mind was confident that my body would obey the instructions of my supra-physical, and the other part was terrified that when I tried to swing the club I should miss the ball completely, or even fall down as my left leg collapsed under me. Perhaps because I knew that if I had to follow the ball into the sand-dunes I should be defeated by the heavy going, and would be unable to climb in and out of bunkers, I kept the ball meticulously on the fairway. For years afterwards Father carried in his note-case a cutting from a national newspaper, "Girl Golf Wonder! Sixteen-year-old player carries off five awards in Hampshire County Championship!"

This is one of the reasons why I know it is exceedingly important to think of one's supra-physical as being in a state of health and efficiency even when its physical counterpart is suffering from the effects of disease, injury, or age. For the supra-physical should, and can, have a most beneficent effect on its carapace; as is frequently demonstrated when its influence produces an apparently "spontaneous" cure after it has received a boost of energy from someone else's supra-physical...the basic principle behind many types of extra-material healing.

The supra-physical can suffer the reverse of this benign process and, if the personalty allows it to do so, can become affected by a resonance to ailments and imperfections which properly should not extend beyond the physical body. This is why it is dangerous to personalize one's maladies. One may not be able to cure the body of its rheumatism or its acne, but there

78

is no point in thinking "MY arthritis" or "MY spots" to a degree which may inflict these miseries on the more subtle components of the personality.

The desire to cling to youth often defeats its own object; for if too much energy is directed towards maintaining a supra-physical which should have been outmoded, the current one becomes depleted, which results in premature ageing. The character is also likely to deteriorate, for this refusal to face reality is no more and no less than a particularly tiresome form of sulk.

Such sulks can even be lethal, as I learned when I was a Roman woman of forty. I was still healthy and handsome; but I found it easier to blame the scribes for writing illegibly than to admit that my eyes were less efficient than they used to be, and I had recently lost three of my excellent teeth. I might not have minded this so much had I not met a much younger man with whom I fell in love, and whom I contrived to see frequently by appointing him as the household physician.

He was dilatory in displaying affection, and each new white hair, each additional wrinkle, reminded me that time was running short. So in the hope that he would realise how much he would miss me if I were to die, I staged an elaborate pseudo-suicide. Having caused a marble sarcophagus to be carved, I invited my acquaintances to a farewell banquet: which was considered mildly eccentric as this was usually done only when the host had decided that honor demanded he should fall on his sword.

Having made a splendid valedictory speech, which moved many of the more tipsy guests to tears, I withdrew to prepare myself for the scene which I confidently expected to be only the prelude to a far more enjoyable act. I arranged myself in my sarcophagus, now filled with warm, scented water and strewn with white rose petals—I remember thinking that after it had served its present purpose it would make a most elegant bath—and then I summoned my physician.

Imperiously I ordered him to open the veins in my wrist: and waited for him to implore me to remain alive, so that he could lavish upon me his passionate devotion. But instead he obeyed me implicitly. I could not have been more horrified had he murdered me in cold blood. Pride would not allow me to tell him to apply tourniquets: so I had to lie there, watching the water turn pink, and then pinker, and then red. At last I shut my eyes, so that he would not see they were blind with rage.

I am exceedingly grateful to him for having had the insight, the compassion, and the moral courage to call my bluff: for he cured me of any temptation again to use this disgusting form of blackmail. But he received the blast of the long-stored fury when I did a spontaneous recall of that episode when drowsing in a far more prosaic bath: for the Roman is again a physician, called Denys Kelsey.

As I have committed suicide, through false pride or in a temper, at least twice, and have deliberately withdrawn from perfectly adequate bodies on three or four other occasions, I know there is no question of being hauled before celestial judges for punishment or condemnation. But what, at least in my experience, invariably happens is that the part of the personality which tried to escape from a particular problem reproduces a similar situation as soon as possible after it reincarnates.

When the aspect of the personality which deals with concepts has made a scapegoat of its physical body, the supra-physical, which has been put to the trouble of providing a new one, is unlikely to find its other partners congenial. Instead of instinct, intuition, and intellect working smoothly together towards a common goal, they indulge in internecine strife which can cause all three of them considerable trouble, for no matter which is temporarily dominant, they will not be at peace until they choose again to integrate.

So it is unrewarding to commit suicide unless the motive is meritorious, as exemplified by Captain Oates walking away into the Arctic blizzard, or the many heroes who have crunched their cyanide capsules rather than risk betraying friends under torture. But I am sure that we should all be prepared to accept full responsibility for expediting our own death when our body is no longer a useful vehicle through which to transmit our personality.

We no longer enjoy the advantages of a culture in which death is recognized as being no more than a particular type of level-shift which every individual has often experienced. Therefore few people are able to die by the simple act of deciding that the time is ripe to do so. Even when this intention has been clearly formulated there is now the risk that it will prove ineffective, because the efforts of the supra-physical to shed its physical particles may be foiled by complicated medical techniques with which it is entirely unfamiliar.

Therefore I think that everyone should be fully informed of the prognosis of any severe illness, and told the real odds against his making an adequate return to health. It is then for him, and no one else, to choose when, and if, he is ready to die. If either Denys or I become crippled to a degree which prevents us giving any further happiness to ourselves or to other people, especially if our condition makes nursing us an unsavory task, we hope that someone will have the charity to provide the means by which we can treat our bodies with the same compassion with which we have treated the bodies of aged or ailing dogs and horses; and release them from further discomforts.

4

THE SUPRA-PHYSICAL IN MEDICINE
by Denys Kelsey

I believe that the concept of the supra-physical body, as Joan has formulated it, contributes to our understanding of the mechanisms involved in a variety of medical phenomena which are by no means confined to psychiatry.

An example of one of these occurred a year or two before I met her. I was talking with Mr. John Baron, the plastic surgeon, about the problems involved in fixing patients in the sometimes curious positions required for the purpose of transferring skin from one region to another, when I recalled a trick performed by a certain stage hypnotist. He would hypnotise members of the audience whom he had invited onto the stage, cause them to assume bizarre postures which would normally be exceedingly uncomfortable, and leave them there while he carried on with the remainder of his act. When mobility was eventually restored to the living statues, they would sheepishly declare that they had kept their position without any conscious exercise of will and without the least discomfort.

It occurred to me that it might be possible to apply the same principle to some of these patients. Mr. Baron replied that he had a case under his care at the moment who might prove a perfect subject for an experiment.

The patient was a young man who, in an accident, had lost the forepart of his right foot. In order to cover the stump of the foot with skin which would withstand a reasonable amount of wear and tear, it was necessary for an area of skin to be brought down to the foot from the abdominal wall. The procedure was going to need five separate operations.

The first step would be to fashion an area of skin on one side of his abdomen into a tube which would remain attached at each end to preserve the blood supply. Then, as soon as it was apparent that the tube was healthly—a matter of a week or two—the next stage would be to free the upper end of the tube from the abdomen and stitch it into a site on the left forearm. Thus, for the next few weeks, while the tube was establishing itself in this position, the patient's arm would be linked to his abdomen by the tube; and during this period it would be vitally important that his arm did not move, for any movement might exert tension upon the tube.

The next stage would be to sever the lower end of the tube from the abdomen and insert it into a second site, on the left wrist. After this operation the patient's arm would be free again, but it would be carrying the tube of skin, looking rather like a large, looping caterpillar. Then, when the tube was clearly thriving in this situation, it would be possible to undertake the next and most crucial stage.

This would involve detaching one end of the tube from the wrist and then having the patient place his left hand in a precise position on the top of his right foot, so that the free end of the tube could be stitched along one margin of the stump. It would then be necessary for the patient to remain in this position for several weeks. For not until the tube had again become well established would it be safe to detach the other end also from the wrist, open the tube up, and apply it to cover the whole of the wounded area.

The patient agreed enthusiastically to the experiment, and so we decided that for the second stage, during which his left forearm would be linked by the tube to his abdomen, we would rely upon post-hypnotic suggestion to fix his arm in position. The effect was remarkable. Not only did the arm maintain its position with complete accuracy, but when it was released, some three weeks later, there was no stiffness whatever in the fingers, wrist, elbow or shoulder.

Encouraged by this, we decided to use nothing but post-hypnotic suggestion at the fourth stage, to fix his hand to his foot. And we were able to tell him that so long as the precise angle at which his hand had been placed on his foot remained unchanged he could move in any way he liked.

Again the technique was astonishingly successful. The hand never budged on the foot, and the patient was perfectly comfortable throughout the whole period. The fact that one hand was stuck to a foot caused him no inconvenience—it scarcely seemed to register on his consciousness. Moreover he developed an astounding agility, and as he could do everything for himself he made minimal demands upon the nursing staff.

But the most gratifying feature became apparent when, after twenty-eight days, the pedicle was deemed fit for the final operation. I hypnotised the patient again, the pedicle was detached from the wrist, and I gave him the signal to unlock himself. Immediately he had full movement in every joint without a trace of stiffness anywhere. He could arch his spine backwards like an acrobat, and he could manipulate a cigarette lighter with the fingers of his left hand. There was simply no need for physiotherapy to overcome the sort of stiffness which would almost certainly have developed after weeks of immobilisation by any mechanical means.

I would not anticipate a similar result on every patient who happened to be a good hypnotic subject. I am sure, in retrospect, that the essential factor responsible for success in this case was the very efficient link this patient had between his supra-physical and his physical bodies. There was another point which, I think, supports this view. As a rule, when two skin surfaces are in contact for a period of weeks, the sweating which occurs between them usually causes the skin to become soggy and unhealthy; but the skin on both the palm of this patient's left hand and on the top of his right foot, was perfectly normal. As sweating is a function which is not under conscious control, I think its absence in this instance can also be attributed to the efforts of the supra-physical body.

The concept of the supra-physical body offers, as Joan has remarked, a credible rationale for the process of so-called "spiritual healing." In this connection the supra-physical may be likened to a magnet that is placed beneath a sheet of paper upon which have been scattered some iron filings. The lines of force travelling between one end of the magnet and the other will draw the filings into a definite pattern and hold them there. Similarly, the energy of the supra-physical maintains the particles which make up the physical body in a definite pattern, but one of function as well as structure. Disease or injury disturb this pattern, and healing represents the efforts of the supra-physical to bring it back to normal. Medicine and surgery in the ordinary sense concentrate on trying to minimise the task which the supra-physical has to perform: perhaps by remedying a lack of some vitamin or hormone or other essential substance; perhaps by giving a drug which makes it impossible for bacteria to proliferate; perhaps by excising a tumour or by fixing some injured part in the most favourable position for healing to occur. But it would seem a rational procedure also to supplement the energy in the supra-physical and I think there is considerable evidence to suggest that this is possible.

My personal experience of healing in this way is not extensive, but I will quote three instances.

One occurred when Joan slammed the door of the car on her left forefinger. The pain was intense and discolouration appeared immediately; I would have expected swelling to occur very soon, and for the finger to be out of action for some days. We happened to be in the depths of the country, so I pulled the car off the road and told Joan to shift level. Then I clasped her finger in my hand and concentrated first on making a vivid mental picture of its anatomy—the skin, the bones, the nerves, the blood vessels. Then I asked her to "Let the pain flow into my hand so that I can throw it away." After some repetitions of this, she declared that her finger was free of pain. At that point I tried to visualise myself literally driving energy into her finger to accelerate the process of healing.

It would be scientifically indefensible to claim that anything happened as a result of my efforts, but the fact is that the finger did not swell, gave her no further pain, and suffered no loss of function.

In the course of writing this book we visited some Swiss friends who live in Berne. As they were also friends of the surgeon Leo Eckmann, I took the opportunity to watch him perform several operations. In the middle of one morning I came back to the house to find that our hostess had just returned from having a wisdom tooth out. The extraction had been unexpectedly difficult, and was performed under a local anæsthetic which had now largely worn off; so, exhausted and in considerable pain, she had gone to bed. Learning that she was allergic to aspirin, I offered to try to help her with hypnosis. She proved an excellent subject and quickly reached a deep state.

I followed the same technique which had apparently helped Joan. I first placed a hand on her cheek and urged her to let the pain flow into my hand so that

I could "throw it away." Then I made a mental picture of the tooth socket with its blood clot in position, and visualised driving energy into it to hasten the healing. Finally, I told her that within a few moments her state would change to one of normal sleep which would last for an hour, and left her.

A little later, Dr. Eckmann arrived at the house. I explained what I had done and, then, since the hour was almost up, we went to see the patient. She awoke as we entered, and the change in her appearance was remarkable. She was completely free of symptoms and felt so full of energy that she insisted upon getting up and resuming her normal programme. She suffered no further discomfort from the extraction, and the socket healed unusually quickly.

This patient's well-being so impressed Dr. Eckmann, that he invited me to attempt to repeat the procedure upon a patient from whom, on the previous day, I had watched him remove the lobe of a lung.

This patient, a man of sixty, was ready to extend to me the supreme confidence he had in his surgeon, and readily entered hypnosis.

I placed my hand on the bandages over his wound, and asked him to let the pain flow into my hand. It was interesting to note that his breathing, quite spontaneously, became deeper. Suddenly he coughed, opened his eyes in astonishment and exclaimed, "But it did not hurt!" Then I made a mental picture of the structures in his chest wall which had been divided during the operation and imagined myself driving in energy. I am told that this patient made an uneventful and unusually rapid recovery.

I must emphasise that these cases carry no scientific weight whatever. The most that can fairly be said is that they support rather than detract from the validity of the concept of transferring energy to the supraphysical body; and innumerable other therapists could relate more impressive experiences of a similar nature.

At present, very little is known about the essence of the factors involved in the interaction between two personalities; but if it were to become generally accepted that there are levels of reality other than the one which can be perceived through the five senses, such matters could become the subject of unprejudiced research. Then, I suspect, laws would be discovered which govern both the transmission and the reception of the energy involved in healing, and orthodox medicine would be enriched by the addition to its armamentarium of techniques which, at present, are too open to charlatanism.

The concept of the supra-physical body as a distinct element of the personality is important to the understanding of reincarnation and will also, I believe, prove valuable in psychiatry in that it may help one to direct therapy more precisely. The point was illustrated by the case of a young man who was suffering from increasing anxiety.

For the first few sessions, Joan and I saw him together. But his story was so rich in the sort of emotional and conceptual material which often underlies this symptom that we did not suspect that an earlier personality might be involved. For this reason I soon continued the therapy without Joan's assistance.

But as the weeks went by, although ventilation and discussion of this material were bringing him certain benefits, such as improved relationships with his family, his anxiety was not diminishing. And then a session occurred in which I had a curious experience.

When I feel uncertain of the direction of the next step during a course of therapy, I sit for some moments with my eyes closed and my body completely relaxed. I find that in this state I very frequently get a "hunch" which quickly proves of value. But on this occasion, instead of a hunch, I got a very vivid mental picture. I saw a young woman, who I knew intuitively was the patient, wearing a blue dress which belonged to a period of at least a hundred years ago. She was sitting in front of a mirror, smiling at herself, and obviously enjoying the reflection of her teeth which were remarkably white and even.

I recalled then that the patient had told me of an incident which had occurred shortly before his anxiety state had started. He had been in a bar where a fight was on the point of breaking out, and a youth had come up to him and said, "I'm going to kick your teeth in!" My patient declared that he was not normally averse to a roughhouse, but these words had caused him literally to feel faint, and he had bolted. He had been ashamed of what he called his cowardice, but also bewildered by it; as he put it: "He was only a little chap—I could have eaten him!"

I regarded this episode as, at most, merely the trigger which had precipitated his illness, and had attached little importance to it. But now, taking into consideration also the fact that the patient's teeth were quite unusually well kept and regular, I realised that it might be of significance. Support for this idea came when I asked him if he often had to visit the dentist. He blushed at the question, and then admitted that the idea of anyone touching his teeth filled him with such repugnance that he had never been near a dentist.

A week later Joan entered the story. At about five o'clock this patient's relatives had telephoned to say that on going into his room that morning they had found him deeply unconscious from a large overdose of sleeping pills. The local doctor, who had been with him most of the day, had just left, satisfied that the danger was over. The patient lived sixty miles from London, and as he was now asleep there was no point in us going down to see him that night. As Joan knew that I would not be free until at least eight o'clock, she decided to do a level-shift alone, to try to find out what had been going on in his mind.

When I went downstairs after my last patient left I was alarmed at what I found, being not yet familiar with the effects on her of a particularly difficult identification. She was obviously in acute pain and tears were pouring down her face. Her mouth was half open, and she managed to tell me that she dared not close it because to do so would increase the agony of her lacerated gums. "I can feel the blood clots in the tooth sockets . . . it was bad enough during the first two days, after he pulled out all her teeth, but then the taste got worse and worse, not only dead blood but pus. Then the fever started . . . and she died on the fourth day. But she forgave him before she died . . ."

It was half an hour, though it seemed infinitely longer, before Joan became sufficiently detached to give a coherent account of what had been happening. She had identified with the woman of whom I had had a mental picture during the last session with the patient more quickly and completely than she had expected to be able to do. The period was the third decade of the nineteenth century, in the county of Somerset in the West of England. The woman was about eighteen and had married a much older man because he was the most prosperous farmer in the district. He was so besotted with his young bride that she was able even to refuse him his marital rights, on the excuse that she was too young to have a baby, which would "spoil her pretty figure." She was renowned for the excellence of her teeth, for at that time scurvy was prevalent and few adults had many teeth left. She enjoyed smiling at young men as much as they enjoyed being smiled on. Her husband's jealousy steadily increased, until one night, in a fury of rage and thwarted sex, he flung her on the bed, and lashed her wrists and ankles to the corner-posts.

Joan thinks his original intention was only rape, and that his wife drove him beyond the brink of sanity by mocking him. He ran to the stables to fetch the pincers which he used for extracting nails from the hooves of his horses. He used this instrument to wrench out all her teeth.

Joan presumed that the patient had been the farmer, and that his reaction to the threat to his own teeth had been based on the fear of retribution for his savagery. She hoped that he would be very much better now that she had relived the experience for him.

By the following evening he had recovered sufficiently from his overdose for his family to bring him to see us. It was immediately apparent that he was no better at all. He was still acutely agitated, and I had no doubt that, given the opportunity, he would repeat his attempt at suicide. I therefore arranged for his admission to a private nursing home.

When we visited him next day he seemed no longer to be suicidal but was still acutely agitated. He repeated the story of that incident in the bar, over and over again, laying particular stress, as though this explained everything, on the fact that the youth had approached him on his right-hand side. Joan told the patient about her level-shift, but the story left him completely unmoved.

At our next visit he launched yet again into an account of the episode in the bar, still laying stress on the fact that, "He came up on my right side, you see!" This reminded Joan that the husband had stood on the right-hand side of the bed; and she realised that the patient had been—not the husband—but the wife. The effect upon the patient of this news was dramatic. He had not the slightest difficulty in accepting the entire story as valid, and by the end of the session his anxiety had vanished.

I did not expect that this degree of improvement, which had occurred so suddenly and, so far as the patient was concerned, so smoothly, would persist. I fully anticipated that by the next morning he would have slipped back, at least a little; but, on the contrary, we found him completely calm and very cheerful. On the following day he was equally well and it seemed unjustifiable to keep him in the nursing home any longer. I telephoned to his family to collect him, warning them that they should remain alert to the possibility of a relapse. However, all this happened more than five years ago, and so far his anxiety has not recurred.

Of the general validity of Joan's ability to shift level and identify with an earlier personality of someone with whom she has a personal link, I have no doubt whatever. Her only mistake in this instance had been to assume that the patient had been the husband. As it was, the fact that he did not react at all to being identified with the husband, but such an immediate and lasting recovery followed identification with the wife, is exceedingly interesting.

If the story had offered him merely a convenient fantasy behind which he could shelter, I think it is virtually certain that he would have relapsed within days or weeks; and unless Joan, by some process which does not fall within the ordinary framework of understanding, had been able to relive the experience on his behalf, I think it is most improbable that he would have recovered without undergoing an intense abreaction himself.

One evening the conversation had turned upon the probable causes of alcoholism. No one had contributed anything original, so after dinner I asked Joan to shift level and see if she could find any relevant information.

She lay down on the sofa, closed her eyes, and in a couple of minutes snapped her fingers to indicate she was ready for the first question.

"What are the causes of alcoholism?" I asked her.

"There are many causes, but one of them is when alcohol has been used as a primitive anæsthetic to dull the pain of an amputation. I am seeing men who have been wounded in a minor battle . . . the period is the Napoleonic wars. They are in a large barn which is being used as an operating theatre . . . there are holes made by cannon fire in the walls. Some of the wounded are lying on straw, the others on the earth floor. A surgeon, holding a bloodstained saw, is leaning against a trestle table, waiting for the next patient to be put on it . . . the surgeon is exhausted.

"The men waiting their turn are trying to drink themselves into oblivion . . . or at least to get drunk enough to numb the pain. But some of them vomit the crude *eau de vie* before it has had time to take effect. The Frenchmen and the 'enemy' . . . I don't know their nationality except that they are not English . . . have tremendous compassion for each other . . . it seems quite irrelevant that they have so recently fought on opposite sides. The stench of gangrene is appalling . . . I shall have to break off for a minute or I shall throw up . . . ."

When she had again shifted level after a brief rest, I repeated my question.

"Now I am seeing one man much more clearly than any of the others. He is in great pain, and in despair because his shattered leg will have to be cut off. He has had some *eau de vie* but not enough to help him . . . he is terrified of screaming when he is carried to the table . . . and of dying of pain. He is watching the leather jug which is being taken from man to man on the other side of the barn. He is praying that it won't be empty before he gets another chance at it . . . . He has an anguished longing for more and more alcohol . . . it is the only hope for dulling his agony. He died of loss of blood while he was still longing for alcohol . . . .

"Someone who has died when longing for alcohol to stop unbearable pain may find that pain reawakens his longing for alcohol . . . but he wants more and more of it, because in the original situation he didn't get *enough* of it to do any good . . . this is the start of the craving."

"How can the condition be cured?"

"In the case of the wounded man take him back to the original situation . . . but be sure he has not taken any alcohol when you do so. It is important that he does not confuse the present with the past. He will be freed only by regressing, unless someone like me can relive it for him and so release the trapped energy. This used to be done by priests, usually by two of them working together. This was so that the two priests could check with each other to be sure that neither had missed any factor, and also because they could share the burden of identification. It is the release of the repressed energy which causes the abreaction . . . either the patient feels it or it is felt by the person who is acting as a priest."

"Can you tell me anything about addiction to morphia?"

"Opium I have known in many lives . . . it was used in very wise civilisations. But it is important to give enough of it. A quarter grain of morphia may arouse a need which it does not satisfy . . . it is the unsatisfied need which leads to the desire for more . . . and so leads to a craving should the person die in acute pain."

"Was opium used for other purposes except the relief of pain?"

"Only by fools!"

There had already been several occasions when Joan, either through a dream or during a level-shift, had produced some specific piece of information which, although it had no relevance to anyone we had yet met, soon proved to have preceded the arrival of a patient to whose therapy it was entirely apposite. I am inclined to think that it was more than a coincidence that soon after the episode of the Napoleonic soldier who had died in agonising sobriety during the amputation of his leg, something very akin to the mechanism of alcoholism she had described was observed in practice.

A young man who was visiting friends nearby came to dine with us one evening. He confided to me that he feared he was becoming an alcoholic, and asked me if I might be able to help him. He had to leave in forty-eight hours which, I pointed out, did not leave us long for therapy. However, he agreed to the suggestion that we might have two preliminary sessions and then, if he felt they were promising, he could return as soon as possible.

He was highly intelligent and rather cynical, and had frankly admitted that he could not accept our theories about reincarnation. I thought he would be difficult to hypnotise, but he reached a deep level very rapidly, and immediately went into a curious spasm. I called for Joan, and by the time she arrived, in a couple of minutes, the spasms had turned to a violent writhing, which affected only his head and trunk. It seemed as though he was struggling to escape from bonds which were holding his arms in a spread-eagled position. He thrust his head back until his spine arched in an extremity of effort. He was making heartrending noises half groan, half cry. In a barely decipherable splutter he gasped, "They are cutting my tongue out . . . with a shiv."

Joan was trying to help him by sharing his experience, but could only get a sketchy outline of the background, as we were both fully occupied in keeping him from falling off the couch. The period was the Spanish Civil War, probably in 1938. He had been working for some kind of resistance movement, or else was taking a message behind the enemy lines . . . he had been caught, and was being tortured to reveal the names of people he was working with. He had been savagely beaten and kicked, which took place in a stone-built hut. The four men who were trying to extract information must have heard something which alarmed them; for they suddenly decided that they must make a fast getaway. They had already trussed his feet together, and they now tied his wrists to iron rings in opposite walls. Cutting out his tongue was an afterthought . . . to make sure that as he would not give his secret away to them he would not be able to tell it to anyone. He died alone, many hours later, agonised not only by pain but by thirst . . . the craving for water becoming more and more predominant. Added to his physical anguish was the fear that his friends would think he had betrayed them by slipping over the border, and would never know that he had refused to divulge their names.

It was very difficult to pull him back to the present day. When I first grasped his hand he identified me with one of his captors and became violent. Gradually I got him to obey such instructions as, "Grasp my hand: release it: grasp it again: let it go: press your hand against the wall." Slowly he reclaimed his present identity and recognised us and his surroundings.

When I believed he was back in normal conscious-ness I told him to move from the couch to a chair. As he did so, he asked for a glass of water. I fetched him a large tumblerful, which he drained and then demanded a second and yet a third. I told him he had drunk as much water as was good for him, but he shouted, "Bring me a jug!"

At this point I realised that he was not completely back in the present, but was still suffering from the thirst in which he had died. I told him to sit on the edge of the couch while I counted slowly from twenty down to one; which brought him fully back into the present. He said, as though startled, "I am no longer in the least thirsty!"

He then told me, for the first time, that for as long as he could remember he had been subject to a compul-sive thirst. Wherever he happened to be, he would be acutely anxious until he had assured himself that he would be able to get something to drink the moment he became thirsty. In a strange house, or in a classroom or cinema, he was ill at ease until he had found out where he could instantly get a glass of water. When he was older and had become introduced to alcohol this too often became the focus of his compulsive need.

Immediately after this session, his compulsion disappeared and in the year which has elapsed he has had no desire for alcohol, and has, in fact, been a teetotaller.

His attitude to this experience is interesting. He admits wholeheartedly that his recovery was due to that one session. But he is still of the opinion that it has no bearing on the validity of reincarnation.

One of the difficulties in psychiatry is that similar symptoms may have very different origins. Take, for instance, the irrational fear of feathers. As Joan has described, in the case of Dr. Kerr-Clarkson this fear had its source in the death of one of his earlier personalities which was associated with vultures. But four years ago a patient of mine, a woman of thirty with an almost identical phobia, was cured of it by reliving an episode in which, at the age of three, she had fallen down in a farmyard and been trampled on by a flock of geese.

If the patient can relive the relevant episode which has occurred in his current lifetime he will probably be cured. But supposing neither the patient nor his relatives can remember such an episode, for the excellent reason that it never occurred: how then can one hope to explain the symptom?

Here we get into the field of psychoanalysis, and begin to think in the terms of the symbolical significance which feathers might have for this particular patient as a result of the tortuous mechanisms of the unconscious. And while there is no doubt that in a certain number of cases this line of search will produce the answer, it is equally certain that in a considerable proportion of cases it will be unsuccessful.

In a proportion of such failures, the cause undoubtedly lies within the patient, who, for one reason or another, is unable to bring himself to face some essential aspect of himself. But this explanation, which is exceedingly tempting to a therapist who is resolutely determined not to countenance the possibility that there may be other levels of the patient's experience in which the answer might lie, can be overdone. Only time and experience will show whether I am right, but I hope that the concept of the supra-physical body will contribute to our understanding of a variety of conditions which, in my experiences may be very difficult to relieve.

For instance, the pain experienced by some people which appears to be coming from a limb that has been amputated; the so-called phantom limb. I recall such a case which I encountered early in my psychiatric career. The patient was a man of fifty with an unusually powerful physique of which he had always been proud. But at the age of fifteen, an injury to a knee had become septic, necessitating, eventually, the loss of that leg. Ever since the amputation he had suffered intense phantom limb pain. Two operations, aimed at freeing any nerves in the stump which might have been caught up in scar tissue, had proved totally ineffective, and two years before he consulted me, he had undergone an operation on his spinal cord at which the nerve tracts carrying pain from that region were cut: but still the pain persisted.

Psychologically, it was not difficult to find personality factors which might, theoretically, have accounted for his pain, but they were dealt with thoroughly, and still the pain was unaffected. It seems at least possible that the original injury to his physical leg was, in this case, for some reason transmitted to his supra-physical, which refused to accept that the leg had been removed, and it is conceivable that therapy directed at healing his supra-physical might have brought relief.

Related to this type of problem, possibly, are some of those cases in which, following an accident, a lack of function persists which is in excess of what the remaining physical disability would seem to justify. Undoubt-edly some of these cases are linked to a hope of finan-cial compensation for the accident on a scale which would be diminished by a complete recovery; but I do not think this explains all of them. It seems to me at least possible that sometimes it is the supra-physical which has been injured and still needs treatment.

Another condition which may be difficult to relieve is hypochondriasis, the fear that one is suffering, or about to suffer, from some grave disease. It is charac-teristic of this type of anxiety that it is not relieved by the most detailed reassurance, based upon the find-ings of searching examination and investigations. A proportion of these cases can be explained and helped along orthodox psychological lines: for instance, their fear may be the expression of unconscious feelings of guilt for which they are trying to punish themselves. But there are others in which this approach seems to be valueless, and in at least some of these, I believe that the anxiety stems from an earlier supra-physical which died of the disease from which the patient is convinced he is still suffering.

Finally, there is the rather large group of cases whose symptoms tend to be labelled "hysterical." Such patients either have a physical symptom for which no organic cause can be found, or an organic condition which appears to be causing a quite disproportionate degree of distress or disability. And these, preeminently, are the patients who tend to be suspected of having symptoms for an unconscious purpose.

Sometimes this suspicion is justified, as in the case of the patient I described in the second chapter who suffered from a paralysis of her legs. In that instance, the purpose was quickly discovered, and as soon as she could see a more acceptable way of dealing with her situation, the use of her legs returned. But there are occasions when the therapist, to his own entire satis-faction, has exposed the patient's unconscious purpose, yet the symptoms still persist. At such times it may be particularly tempting to assume that the patient prefers to continue to be ill. Undoubtedly, in certain instances, this assumption is well founded; but very often, I believe, it is grossly unjust to the patient, because his symptoms, like those of some of the sufferers from hypochondriasis, are a resonance to an earlier supra-physical.

Two examples of this mechanism were furnished by Joan. Obviously they would have been more telling if they had concerned patients who had no knowledge of our ideas; but if Joan's faculties enable her to recognise a mechanism in herself, it will be easier to recognise when it is occurring in other people.

The first occasion was when I decided to try to find out why Joan, when reading or eating in bed, always lay flat on her back, her legs out straight and only raising her head a few inches from her single pillow. This worried me, because of the obvious danger of choking when swallowing in a supine position. I also knew that she had already scalded herself severely enough to be kept in bed for ten days and scarred on the neck and chest for several months, when her thumb had slipped off the handle of a mug of nearly boiling soup. Whenever I reminded her to sit up she did so, but when alone would revert absentmindedly to her habitual position. Matters came to a head one day when I found her drenched in orange juice. Suddenly I realised that her posture reminded me of that of a patient who is paralysed from the waist down. I mentioned this to her and she told me of an incident which had occurred when she was four years old.

She had been running ahead of her nanny to open a massive oak door at the end of an avenue in her parents' garden. But the door had been taken off its hinges for repair, and had been left propped temporarily in position by a plank. The plank had slipped when Joan touched it. She remembered the door falling towards her, trying to run, being knocked down by a blow between her shoulder blades, and then lying trapped, face downwards. A gardener had tried to lift the door off her, but it was so heavy that he could not do so until two other men arrived to help him.

The nanny lifted her up, and when Joan said her leg was hurting, the nanny, who must have panicked, stood her on it to see if it was broken. It was: Joan felt it crumple under her, and then she fainted.

She retained a vivid memory of the difficulties in the healing of this fracture, which had necessitated her leg being kept in plaster for many months. But she had no recollection of a fact about which she had later been told—that for three weeks it was feared that she would be paralysed. As her fourth and fifth thoracic vertebrae still show signs of an old fracture, I presume her spinal cord had been bruised.

When I asked Joan to shift level I anticipated that she would recover details of this period of paralysis. But instead of regressing to her childhood she found herself identified with a girl of twenty who had been paralysed from the waist down in a riding accident.

This girl was an earlier personality of her own. Her Christian name was Lavinia, she was English, and died in 1875. She was married, but not to me.

As by this time I was familiar with hearing Joan reliving episodes from earlier lifetimes as matter-of-factly as though she were telling me about some incident from her current one, I was startled when she exclaimed, "Bring me back fast! I am getting so closely identified with Lavinia's paralysis that I'm afraid it's affecting my own legs."

In a couple of minutes she had returned to normal-waking-consciousness—but she could not move her legs. This was a new and most alarming experience for her, but she remained sufficiently detached to tell me to put my hand on her back to discover which muscles were out of action.

Although I was already familiar with the concept of the supra-physical body, I was not yet fully alive to the importance, for treatment, of distinguishing between it and other aspects of the personality. Therefore I told her to shift level again to try to find out more about the circumstances of the accident. She did this in considerable detail, the essential information being that Lavinia had been locked in her bedroom by her husband to prevent her riding to hounds on that particular morning. His motive was jealousy, because she had danced too often with a young man whom she had met for the first time at a hunt ball the previous evening, and her husband was determined she should not meet him again.

Lavinia had climbed out of the bedroom window and so reached the stables, only to find that all the horses were out except a young stallion that even her husband dared not ride. She saddled him with the aid of a reluctant stable-boy, who cannot have tightened the girths properly; for when she was in sight of the hounds, rebellious and triumphant, the sidesaddle slipped as she was taking a fence, and both she and the horse suffered a heavy fall which broke her back.

As I assumed that it was Lavinia's anger against her husband which had caused her to fail completely to integrate, I concentrated for some hours on trying to bring every facet of such feelings to the surface. This approach had no beneficial effect whatever and Joan's legs were still useless. Finally she said, "Lavinia's body will never be able to go until you have healed it."

The idea of healing an earlier supra-physical had never previously occurred to me, so I had to act intuitively. Turning Joan onto her face, and telling her to shift level so as to be receptive, I placed my hands on her back in the region which, I hoped, corresponded with the site of Lavinia's fracture. Then I made a vivid mental picture of such an injury, telling Joan that I was going to drive energy through her body into the supraphysical of Lavinia.

102

I have noticed that when attempting any kind of healing, I feel on some days that I am being more effective than on others, and there is also a sensation that, for the time being, I have done all I can. I experienced this after about ten minutes, and told Joan that Lavinia's fracture was now healed and that she would find that she had now regained the full use of her legs. Soon she was able to move them, albeit rather feebly. I then told her to return to the present day and normal-waking-consciousness. We both assumed that this was the end of the incident, for her legs were soon functioning normally.

However, the following morning she told me that during the night she had found it difficult not to resonate to Lavinia and had twice woken to find that she was suffering a recurrence of the paralysis. But as these symptoms had subsided after she had switched on the light and read for a few minutes she had decided not to waken me.

That afternoon I again sat beside her while she shifted level. Again she identified closely with Lavinia, and we learned many more details about the three years she had been confined as a cripple, either to her bed or to a chaise-lounge in her bedroom. There was a recurrence of the previous session's symptoms, so I repeated the same technique. Suddenly Joan exclaimed, "Now I can see Lavinia getting up from her bed and walking freely. There is no need to do any more!" She then fell peacefully asleep, and slept until early the next morning.

Thereafter Joan no longer assumed her supine posture, and now alters her position as spontaneously and frequently as would anyone else with normal powers of movement. But there was another feature which I found equally interesting.

The first Lavinia session had ended when I told Joan that the injury suffered by her earlier supra-physical had been healed, and that therefore she would be able to use her legs normally. But the fact that she had again resonated to Lavinia during the following night, with a recurrence of symptoms, indicates that the return of function had been due only to my suggestion.

By contrast, the second session had ended when Joan herself declared that she could see Lavinia moving freely: and after this there was no relapse.

So it seems reasonable to conclude that something was achieved in the second session which had a validity of its own, was not merely due to my suggestion, and affected Lavinia at least as much as it affected Joan.

A year or so after this episode, Joan was bitten on the corner of her left eye by a mosquito. There was considerable swelling and some discolouration, but nothing which would not have cleared up in a couple of days without recourse to antibiotics. She told me that she was feeling a degree of pain and alarm which was entirely disproportionate, and that as she had suffered the same exaggerated reaction to a mosquito bite which affected her eye on several other occasions she wanted me to do something about it. She added that mosquito bites on any other part of her body were never more than mildly annoying, and that when working with her father in his Mosquito Control Institute she had often given mosquitoes blood meals from her arm as part of her job as his laboratory assistant.

Within a couple of minutes of shifting level, she said, "I died of an insect bite. That is why I am so frightened. He was an Egyptian captain, about twenty-five years old. He was bitten on the eyelid while he was asleep . . . by a fly, not by a mosquito. His face is terribly swollen, and covered with suppurating scabs.... I think he must have septicæmia."

She was becoming distressed, so I told her that I would perform on her face the sort of surgical toilet which I would have performed on the face of the Egyptian captain. Then, taking a piece of moist cotton wool, I began gently to swab her forehead. Suddenly she announced, "You are not doing it the right way. You should have two pieces, and swab outwards from the centre so that there is no smearing."

I carried out her instructions, while her degree of identification increased. "I am in a torment of anxiety . . . if I die my men will be left without a leader. I am trying to force my brow and cheek apart with my fingers in order to see the little crack of light which tells me I am not blind . . . ."

Then suddenly, in her normal voice, "You should be doing that with water and a white linen cloth."

I fetched a small bowl of water and one of her white linen handkerchiefs, which I wrung out and laid on her forehead. "No! It must be kept moving!"

At this point I set myself to make a clear mental picture of a face in the condition she had described, and visualised myself performing a meticulously careful toilet upon it. After about ten minutes, she said, "That is much better . . . but you have missed some of the scabs. There are some still left under my hair and in my nostrils." I attended to these, and soon she said, "There are no scabs left now.... He is healed.... He was a fine-looking man. . . . But there is still something wrong with him . . . . There is a hole in his skull . . . . One of his comrades must have trephined him!"

I put my hand on her head at the place she indicated and visualised the wound closing. After a few minutes, she gave a deep sigh of relief and said, "Everything is all right now." And fell peacefully to sleep.

When she woke, after three hours, she had no further pain or apprehension, and the swelling of her eye had practically subsided.

When we come to look back on these two episodes in some years' time, my efforts of treatment may seem somewhat naïve and crude. But I think the concept of trying to heal an earlier supra-physical may be seen to have contained the seed of a contribution to the treatment of a variety of conditions. As so many psychiatrists have been moved to exclaim, "Insight is not enough!" Insight does not necessarily imply cure, and this is understandable. For if the symptom is coming from a source which, on its own level, is as real as a stone in the shoe, and a great deal more dynamic, relief will depend not on the mere recognition of its presence, but on its removal.

The supra-physical body became for me an almost tangible reality on the 4th of February 1960, when Joan was undergoing a small exploratory operation. The procedure itself was trivial but the issue at stake was not, so it was a time of considerable anxiety. I had accompanied her in the elevator to the operating theatre and remained with her while Pentothal was injected. Immediately she was unconscious I returned to her room as she had previously asked me to do. I was sitting in the armchair, thinking of her very intensely, when I felt her come and sit on my knee. Never before had I realised that anything immaterial could seem so solid!

I "knew" she was telling me to get a pencil and some paper. I did so and returned to the chair. Then Joan began to "dictate."

There was no sensation of a voice talking to me, but ideas were being communicated as directly as though by speech. The material concerned a patient who had just come under our care and was soon to prove exceedingly relevant. I was kept writing at full speed for some twenty minutes, and then a nurse came in to prepare the bed for the patient's return. Just as positively as I had felt Joan settle on my knee, now I felt her leave.

5

THE CULTIVATION OF THE SENSES
by Joan Grant

The role of the body, both physical and supra-physical, is to increase the range and quality of sensory perception, thereby increasing the field of choice and the capacity to choose benignly. The part the body plays in the evolution of the individual is no less important than the part played by other components of the personality, for no component can develop at the expense of another. Having in my time fallen prey to the delusion that "the great spirit burns the body to the rind," and having therefore wasted a lot of energy in futile asceticism, I know that it is exceedingly misguided to neglect the task of cultivating the five senses.

The majority of adults have allowed their sense of taste to become virtually atrophied, which is particularly foolish, for they thereby discard the personalised diet sheet, compounded of the experience acquired in many earlier bodies, which would have advised them what, and what not, to eat. An intelligent appetite, as opposed to the appetite which has been thwarted and so reacted with gluttony, is one of the most valuable allies to physical health.

The fact that the food served in highly organised communities is likely to look but not taste like the dish it purports to be, is a result, not the cause, of the prevalence of pallid palates. Modern processing has discovered ways of preventing chemical and bacteriological deterioration, but has not been able to keep food "alive" in the sense of being able to retain its supraphysical energy. A corpse can remain unchanged indefinitely if kept at a sufficiently low temperature—a mammoth disclosed by a melting glacier was served as the main course of a Russian banquet at the end of the nineteenth century—but the supra-physical component lingers only briefly after death, and it is this more subtle constituent in our diet which most of us now lack.

The importance of cultivating the sense of taste, not only for pleasure but for protection, is why I consider there are few more repellent sights than a child being cajoled or bullied into eating something he is instinctively trying to reject. If instead he were offered a selection of suitable types of food, and allowed to choose how much, or how little, his body wanted at that particular moment, he would be very much healthier, and the attendant adult far less jaded at the end of the meal. Parents who feel impelled to shovel prescribed amounts of food into their protesting young would have done better to invest in an automobile than in a baby; for they would have done no harm to the machine by rigidly following the manual which advised the correct quantities of oil and gasoline.

The contrast between the taste-education of the average American or English infant, and the robust appetite encouraged in their French contemporaries, especially in rural areas, is illustrated by an episode which Charles and I witnessed in 1956.

The scene is the Hotel Beau Rivage, near Cahors, on the river Lot. We are just finishing our first course when there enters a party of four adults and seven children. The eldest child is about eight years old and the youngest is a baby. While the soup is being served to them the baby wakes up and stares fixedly at the tureen which is in the centre of the table. Mother, who has been preparing a bottle for him by mixing powdered milk with hot water from a thermos, exclaims, "Look! Look! At last Philibert has noticed what we are eating!"

Everyone at the table joins in the excitement. "Philibert must have some soup in his bottle," clamour the other children. "He wants it! He wants it!"

Mother, delighted, tips away half the formula and tops up the bottle with soup—good rich soup it is too, not the pallid broth which is all Philibert could have hoped for if he had been born English or American. He has a good long suck at it, after Mother has enlarged the hole in the teat by prodding it with a hairpin. Then he gazes round and loudly burps his approval.

Halfway through the bottle Philibert is handed to Father, so that Mother can get at her soup before it grows cold. Father, knowing the drill, has emptied his plate quickly. By the time Philibert demands a second helping, the soup tureen has been taken away, so he is given a fragment of truffle omelette. For a moment he is doubtful about the taste of truffle, then chortles with approval.

He is now drowsy, and is handed from lap to lap round the table, a cosy variant of the doormouse at the Mad Hatter's Tea Party in *Alice in Wonderland*. He has nearly completed the circuit when he becomes sufficiently alert to enjoy bread crumbs soaked in the chicken's luscious sauce, which is affectionately fed to him by his eldest sister. Then Philibert, no doubt happily aware that he has laid the foundations of an admirable digestive system, goes serenely to sleep.

Everyone is enchanted, including the occupants of the other tables, who beam or nod to show that they have noticed that yet another Frenchman has graduated from the drab business of mere eating to the appreciative enjoyment of appetite.

From the age of two, I was also given every opportunity of cultivating my appetite, for I had my lunch with the grown-ups, a rare privilege in my generation. I had already learned to eat fast and knew that the smallest smear on my face or even slightly sticky fingers would mean being sent from the room in disgrace. In those lavish days, before the first World War, we had a French chef called René to whom I was devoted. One day I was assisting him to prepare a *julienne* of vegetables—so kind a man he was that he never let me guess how much I hindered—when I stretched out my hand too far across the choppingboard, too fast for him to withhold the flashing knife. The top joint of my left fore-finger hung by a sinew. I screamed and René fainted.

Luckily a doctor who was staying in the house did such an excellent repair that I now have only a faint scar, but René took the accident far more hardly than I did. Every night, after I was in bed and my current governess had gone to her solitary supper, he brought offerings to me: chocolate rabbits stuffed with cream, marzipan birds perched on spun-sugar nests, patés of crab, rich morsels of duck mousse; banquets in miniature on which I thrived.

I had always thought that this early training had been the foundation of the highly developed sense of taste which makes it easy for me to detect the ingredients in a dish, and so to be able to reproduce it. But I only recently discovered that the faculty was acquired much earlier in my long-history. I had apologised for a deficiency in the soup, which no one else seemed to have noticed; and that same evening, while I was doing a level-shift to find out some other information, someone asked me the question, "When did you acquire your hyper-acute sense of taste?"

To my surprise I found that the answer came from a life of which I had had no previous knowledge. I belonged to a nomadic tribe whose diet was mainly vegetarian: I cannot recall whether this was due to the scarcity of game or their lack of expertise as hunters.

Before any newly discovered plant was officially declared edible it was tested by the tribal taster. He, for I was then male, put a minute fragment of the unfamiliar leaf or fruit or fungus, first on and then under his tongue, concentrating intently on his reactions to it. If the taste were agreeable he would swallow a larger morsel; and then, during the next few days, would ingest increasingly large amounts until he was sure that even a belly-full produced no unfavourable side effects. When side effects occurred their nature was given careful consideration. Were these so slight that the substance could be used as food in an emergency? Had they some specific effect, such as to cause profuse sweating, or purging, or to alter the rate of heartbeat or respiration, which indicated that they might be a valuable addition to the tribal medicine?

I believe that the reason why many primitive peoples have a remarkable knowledge of plants which can be used as herbal remedies is due not to chance observation, but to this type of specific training. Gypsies, for instance, were well aware of the efficacy of a preparation of foxglove leaves as a palliative for dropsy and certain heart conditions long before a gypsy woman told her secret remedy to a nineteenth-century doctor through whom it was introduced, as digitalis, into the pharmacopœia.

The medieval taster, who took a mouthful from every dish before it was offered to his master, worked under rather easier conditions. He was always told exactly what ingredients had been used in its preparation, and so, although this was difficult enough if the sauce were highly spiced, he only had to detect the presence of an alien substance. This ability was essential to his profession, for if he had had to wait until symptoms of poisoning developed, his employer would have gone supperless to bed.

If a child, or even an adult, has allowed his tastebuds to fall into disuse these can still be reeducated. Among the children who lived at Trelydan during the war were several who were alleged to suffer from very delicate digestions. In each case the mother, faced with the dual anxiety of a husband on active service and the responsibility of looking after her own children, because nanny was now doing war work, had become far too concerned with what they should or should not eat. The complexity of the diet-sheets they brought with them was enough to show me that fear, not food, was the cause of their indigestion: fear that if they did not eat what they were given they would "never grow up to be a man like Daddy"; fear they would be ill if they so much as nibbled some forbidden delicacy.

As I never accepted a junior guest except at "owner's risk" I tore up the diet-sheet as soon as the escort had left, and told the new arrival that he was now free to eat as much or as little as he wished of anything which happened to be available. All but two were delighted at this unexpected freedom, and willingly accepted my rider that the new regime would begin the moment they had proved their ability to throw-up at will. This useful art came in very handy when a couple of them ingested an enormous quantity of unripe plums, for they were able to get rid of the load at the first twinge of discomfort instead of risking a painful colic.

But one little girl was most indignant when she found I had no intention of "tempting" her to eat. In considerable dismay she watched me calmly removing her untouched supper tray, and then wailed, "My mummy will be very angry with you if you don't make me drink my milk!"

"Your tummy knows better than Mummy what it needs," I said consolingly. I patted her round little stomach, and added, "Look how plump and happy it is ... you needn't eat for a week if you don't want to, and it won't mind a bit." She was a warmhearted child, and a few days later thanked me for showing her that meals could be fun.

Another child, a boy of eight, was even more outraged when he found that no one took any notice when he sat through a meal without eating a mouthful. He followed me out of the dining-room and shouted, "When I starve to death I hope you get hanged!"

He kept up his hunger strike for three days, and I found it difficult not to show I was worried. The other children comforted me with assurances that he was only being tiresome, and told me that he had boasted that I would soon behave just like his mother and start imploring him to eat. As they despised the ploy of bullying the grown-ups by evoking needless anxiety, they added to his problems by discovering his secret cache of biscuits and removing it. Deprived of a familiar adult target he then started to bully a smaller child by rubbing axle-grease on her head, which reduced her to tears as her hair was curly and would now be very difficult to wash.

At this point, Gillian and two other teen-agers decided to take a hand in the treatment. They took off his clothes, smeared him all over with mouldy jam and flung him into a nettle bed. Whether being on the other end of the stick was a retribution he had long been seeking, or whether the exercise of extricating himself from the nettles gave him an irresistibly strong appetite I do not know. But he enjoyed an excellent lunch and thereafter tucked in as enthusiastically as any of the others. The children warmly accepted him after this episode, for he had undergone these reprisals, which were long overdue, without resentment, and had neither whined nor sneaked. He became both affectionate and a great credit to their forthright therapy.

The experiment of letting the intake of children be decided solely by their instinct and appetite took place over twenty years ago, and it is encouraging that none of them have since suffered any form of digestive ailment. Even more rewarding is the fact that these children's children, brought up with the same freedom of choice, have shared this benign immunity.

Probably because the senses of taste and smell are so closely linked, I have a nose whose efficiency would do credit to a spaniel. Denys first had evidence of its range when we were walking in a park near our first home in Highgate Village, on an evening when the air was heavy with gasoline fumes and London fog. I suddenly stopped, sniffling alertly, and exclaimed, *"Chimonanthus Fragrans* . . . how very odd!" He looked bewildered, so I added, "But it *is* odd to find it in a park . . . and flowering in November." Following the scent, along the path and through a sooty shrubbery, I saw, twenty feet from the ground and nearly smothered by laurels, a single spray of the flowers whose fragrance I had so instantly identified.

A nose can not only be a source of pleasure but can provide useful information. Like most other animals, I can smell fear, which has an entirely specific smell, musky and slightly acrid. This can be a helpful clue when trying to decide whether someone's off-beat behaviour is motivated by aggression or only by acute anxiety. A discrete sniff will often tell one more about a patient's progress than will a glance at his temperature chart; and some diseases have a characteristic smell which can be an important aid to diagnosis.

An example of the diagnostic angle occurred while I was recording a life as a strolling player in the country now called Italy. I, Joan, was in my London house in the summer of 1938. The woman I used to be, whose name was Carola, was in the stable loft of an inn, a few days walk from Perugia, in the summer of 1526. Carola was then aged sixteen and was nursing a woman called Lucia through smallpox.

The identification of the recall was so complete that I became nauseated by the stench of Lucia's disease

114

and on several occasions had to break off dictation and run to the bathroom to vomit. The description of what I was recording was so painfully detailed that my secretary suffered the same reactions, and she was in the bathroom when the doorbell rang.

The stranger on the doorstep identified himself as a doctor, who had come to visit a friend who was convalescing with me after an operation. He looked at me quizzically, and said, "I suggest you let me have a look at you before I go up to see my patient . . . for you're extraordinarily pale."

Being still more or less on two levels at once, instead of dissembling I said frankly, "There's nothing the matter with me. I have been reliving a sixteenth-century smallpox, and the smell is so disgusting that I can't get it out of my nose."

He accepted my statement calmly: put down his bowler hat and umbrella and followed me into the drawing room. He then asked me to describe the signs and progress of the disease; which I proceeded to do, with a wealth of unsavoury detail which I deleted from the published version.

When I had finished, he told me that my description of each stage of the disease, and its duration, had been remarkably accurate. And that the only point on which he could fault me was when I claimed that smallpox had a specific and unforgettable smell.

"But it has! I can still smell it!" I exclaimed with some heat.

To which he replied soothingly, "I am not denying that there would have been attendant disgusting smells, especially when the patient was being nursed under such primitive conditions. But there is no diagnostic one. I can state this categorically, for I have recently returned from India, where I spent two years as the medical officer in charge of the smallpox wards of a large hospital."

I did not see him again for six weeks. This time he

came to show me an article in a medical journal which had come in that morning's post. It described a rare type of smallpox, which had been rampant in Europe during the Middle Ages but was now almost unknown. A sentence had been underlined in red ink by the doctor, "This type of smallpox can easily be distinguished from all other types: for the patient exudes a specific stench which once smelt can never be confused with any other."

Although the smell of disease is instructive it is unpleasant, but the smell of a healthy body is endearing, especially the smell of a body which one's own finds congenial: adult bodies, children's bodies, animals' bodies—even the body of a baby, providing it is free from an undertone of regurgitated milk. The smell of sweat is in no way repulsive providing it is fresh; but it soon turns rancid, and it is the smell of yesterday's sweat on clothes which causes the purveyors of deodorants to prosper. The manner in which the majority of people have allowed themselves to be deprived of the pleasure latent in their nostrils is exemplified by the notion that the best they can hope for is to smell of nothing at all.

If the natural range of auditory perception is comparable to a full orchestra, most people hear only thuds from the drum or blasts from the trumpet. If our ears are constantly being assaulted by the shriek of brakes, the insistence of telephone bells, the parrot-house screech of voices in competition, it is only too easy to believe that all sound is potentially hostile.

The cacophony of over-population has led to a society starved of silence. And it is a truism as well as a cliché that one needs silence in order to hear oneself think. The practice of wearing earplugs to shut noise out during sleep soon defeats its object. For the body relies on its ears to act as watchdogs, and when deprived of these natural guardians is likely to demand

116

that the supra-physical aspects of the personality remain in attendance, which results in a shallow doze or insomnia instead of the far more refreshing process of a true level-shift. This situation is in no way improved by the body being bludgeoned into apparent insensibility by barbiturates.

An even more prevalent way of trying to cope with noise is to leave the radio or record player going full blast until the eardrums are so exhausted by this battery that they become ineffective, even to the point of deafness. Another motive for this practice, especially among the young, is that having failed to develop their other sensory resources they have come to rely on a constant stream of noise to assure themselves that they exist. A baby gains self-confidence by finding he can make a noise other than by screaming: by shaking his rattle, or by banging his playpen with a wooden toy: I think the same mechanism causes infantile adolescents to be comforted by the fact that they can produce even louder sounds by flipping a switch or dropping a coin into a jukebox.

One way to find the benison of silence, or at least comparative silence, when living in a city is to wake in the small hours of the night. When Denys and I lived in London, in a house on a very noisy street, I habitually woke at about 3:30 A.M., when my ears could listen to small sounds acutely, which I believe is an exercise exceedingly beneficial in maintaining a fully effective sense of hearing. I found myself instinctively waking at this same hour when we were in a hotel on Madison Avenue. Another useful auditory exercise is to listen intently to orchestral music, at first only following a theme, and then a single instrument, such as a clarinet or flute.

In the country it is much easier to train one's ears, for small sounds are clearly delineated against a back cloth of quietness. The sough of wind in the grass, the sibilant movement of a leaf, the plink of a toad, a note

117

quite distinct from the reply from another toad further down the valley. With very little practice one can literally feel one's eardrums vibrating, and they become lively instead of mere passive receptors of sound.

A friend who was staying with us at our home in France commented that there seemed to be very few birds near the house. As there was a nightingale, two cuckoos, a nuthatch, several sparrows, tree-creepers, blackbirds, and jays, singing within fifty yards, and a woodpecker was hammering the bark of the walnut tree under which we were sitting, I presumed he was very deaf. I thought he might be able to recover his hearing if we could discover its supra-physical cause, so I embarked on a reminiscence which I thought would be a tactful lead, saying that I too had been deaf for three months, after a fractious patient had boxed my ear and totally destroyed the drum. (To the ear specialist's amazement, it recovered completely: he showed me my case history on which he had written, "Chances of recovery. Nil.")

Instead of being comforted by my ready sympathy, my companion looked displeased, and said coldly, "I cannot imagine why you think I am deaf: I happen to have unusually efficient hearing."

So I told him to listen. "But there is nothing to listen to . . ." Then he paused, and exclaimed, "But there are dozens of birds! Now I can see them, too! And the woods are resounding with cooing and cawing . . . and I have never noticed even a pigeon or a rook since I came here!"

Thereafter he woke himself at sunrise so as not to miss the dawn chorus.

The average person uses his eyes only to supply him with essential information: he uses them to read, to drive a car, to dodge buses, but he very seldom really looks at anything.

Teaching a child, or even a grown-up, to use his eyes

is enormously rewarding. The joys of exploring a rock-pool have been described in many autobiographies, but a few square yards of an ordinary meadow can provide material for hours of observation . . . probably at least fifty different kinds of leaves, and a number of engaging insects and beetles. "What have you seen today?" is a question which should evoke an increasingly rich and varied response, and the person who is too purblind to notice what his eyes could have shown him, whatever his age, should be told that he is therefore infinitely more boring than he need be.

Anyone who drives through beautiful scenery, so intent on getting to his destination as quickly as possible that he is aware of nothing except road signs, and the car in front which he is trying to pass, should be made to realise that he is not only depriving himself of pleasure, but demonstrating his inadequacy as a companion. Nothing is more damping than to travel, even along a familiar road, with someone whose response is always, "I didn't notice."

I was walking with two friends recently when I stopped to watch an ant's nest. I was crouching on my haunches, so as to get a closer view of a complicated bridging operation which was being carried out with remarkable speed and cooperation, when one of my companions asked anxiously whether I was feeling faint. They had not even noticed the ants!

However they got the message, and handed it on. The next time we went to stay with them, their son, aged four, was lying face downwards on the lawn. His mother called to him, and he looked up only long enough to whisper, "Shoosh! I am very busy watching my beetle." His parents said that instead of often being bored and constantly demanding new toys he was now able to amuse himself for hours by finding fresh things to look at.

The country child has an unending range of things to discover, providing he has been put on the track of doing so, but the town child has equal if different opportunities for enjoying his vision. When Gillian was less than two years old we discovered the Museum Game, through having been driven into the Victoria and Albert by a sudden downpour when on our way for a walk in Hyde Park. I was wondering how best to exercise her and hoping to find a deserted gallery where we could play hide-and-seek round the showcases, when she suddenly stopped, and pointing at a wax figure, one of about a dozen displaying historical costumes, said, "What kind of chair did that woman sit on?"

The clothes were of the Queen Anne period, so we went to the gallery of eighteenth-century furniture. I expected Gillian's interest to wane after a few minutes, but instead she studied the different types of chairs with the absorbed interest of an antiquarian. Our heroine had by now been named Mary Anne, and having chosen her chair we paid the same attention to selecting the furniture in which she could keep her clothes, a walnut lowboy and a bow-fronted chest. And then added a desk at which she could write her letters.

Many times we returned to the V and A; because Gillian wanted to see the knives and forks Mary Anne ate with, the candlesticks for her table, the embroideries which would have occupied her leisure, the musical instruments she played, the carriage she rode in to visit her friends. Sometimes I only kept one jump ahead of her expanding interest by looking up the relevant facts in the London Library. We discovered the food Mary Anne served to her guests, how it was cooked, how many servants she kept and their various duties, and where she went for her holidays.

We learned still more about her by visiting Kew Gardens, and looking at the flowers she would have grown in her borders. This was easy, for I only had to consult *Sanders Encyclopedia of Gardening* which lists plants indigenous to England, the date on which they were first introduced and their familiar as well as their botanical names. Angel's Tears, Love-in-the-Mist, and Hare's Ear are far easier to remember, and much more evocative, than *Narcissus Triandrus Albus, Nigella,* and *Bupleurum!*

Without for a moment feeling that she was being "educated" Gillian gained a wide-angled view not only of an earlier century but of many related subjects. It gave her the ability to correlate information, to fit each item of data into a much larger framework, which made her later scholastic education exceedingly easy.

I cannot stress hard enough how important it is for children to have their senses developed far younger than is usually considered practicable. The demand for the same story to be read over and over again is not prompted by a desire for it to be repeated, but because the child is starved for fresh books, fresh stories, fresh pictures to stimulate his imagination. The only exception I found to this was when Gillian, aged four, insisted that the same Little Grey Rabbit book should be read to her five evenings running. She then took it from my hand and said, "Now I will read to you for a change"; and to my amazement did so, without getting a word wrong.

She had just reached the final page when her father came into the room and I said, "Isn't Gillian clever, she can actually read . . . and I didn't know she had even learned the alphabet."

She repeated the performance and he too was impressed. We were congratulating her, when she suddenly burst into giggles, turned a somersault on her bed and shouted, "But how can you both be so silly! Of course I can't read yet.... I just learned the book by heart as a joke."

Pictures can be far more interesting even to a small child than picture books, especially if these are made the focus of an impromptu story, either made up by the child herself or told in a way which will capture her interest. The interest which a four-year-old child can take in something apparently as unexciting as someone else's family portraits was shown by Gillian saying to a hostess, "The woman in the blue dress in the drawing room here has much prettier flowers in the posy she is holding than she has in the picture of her in the dining room in your other house." Her hostess, intrigued that Gillian had noticed that there were in fact two portraits, for she had only once been to luncheon in the other house and that was several months previously, said, "The flowers are exactly the same; both portraits were painted by Peter Lely but the other one is an identical copy."

"Then he must have got tired of doing the same thing twice and done different flowers," said Gillian stoutly, "for the flowers *are* different. The other one has got a red rose-bud instead of a pink one, and there are forget-me-nots . . . and a white flower I don't know the name of . . . .

The conversation ended in the three of us driving fifty miles to settle the argument: Gillian's observation proved to be right.

The sense of touch is cultivated by the blind, and by those who follow professions such as surgery or sculpture, but in the majority of people it is the most grievously neglected of all the five senses. Yet in many ways it is the most important, for it can transmit the vital energy of affection.

From infancy, most of us are deprived of the identification provided by skin to skin contact—although this is sometimes prescribed for delicate babies, under the chilling heading of T.L.C. "Tender Loving Care." Very few children have the natural solace of being caressed in mutual nakedness even by their parents: so it is not in the least surprising that they grow up with such a pressure of unsatisfied longing that they try to assuage it during adolescence by premature and pitifully ineffectual sexual experiments. Ineffectual because it is not sex they really crave; it is the physical affection which, as their body-memory of more kindly cultures is constantly reminding them, is their natural right.

To test the validity of this statement, try to communicate with an animal without touching it. Continue talking to your dog, walking your dog, feeding your dog, but refrain from touching him and allowing him to touch you and see what happens. At first he will be bewildered, and then, presuming that you are angry with him, he will produce symptoms of guilt. Continue with this experiment even for a day, and the dog, according to his character, will either mope, or whine, or snarl at you, or run away. I believe that by failing to give our children the comfort and reassurance that we still give to our animals we cause them to follow the same pattern of reactions: they mope, or whine, or snarl at us, or run away to join the lonely hordes of juvenile delinquents.

The modern child seldom suffers from clothes which cause its flesh to cringe in disgust as did the children of my generation. The harsh wool combinations, the starched petticoats and drawers, whose goffered frills felt sharp as razors, the elastic which cut a ridge under our tender chins to clamp huge hats onto our sensitive scalps, are no longer standard tortures. But babies still have to endure the horrid impediment of woolly gloves and become entangled in woolly shawls, and are unlikely to have the freedom of nakedness for which their skin hungers.

I think the least one can do for children is to let them run about naked whenever they like, as did all the children who lived at Trelydan. This not only gives them a much better posture, because the body which is allowed its natural freedom has an innate dignity, but spares them the psychological hazards which can arise from the implication that there is something "nasty" about nakedness. At one time I had nine children living with me, six males and three females, whose ages ranged from seven to seventeen. They wore clothes only when it was necessary to conform with other people's conventions, or to protect themselves from cold or brambles. They shared baths with each other and with my husband and me; I often found two or three of them curled up in bed together like puppies in a basket, but in spite of the gloomy predictions of my acquaintances there were no sexual complications whatever.

It was interesting how quickly visiting adults adapted themselves to these natural conditions. I well remember a Methodist minister from the Middle West, who spent a few days with us on his way home from a mission to Africa. I met him in a train, and finding that his knowledge of English geography was sketchy, for he was hoping to see Loch Lomond, the Lorna Doone country and Shakespeare's birthplace in forty-eight hours, an impractical ambition without a helicopter, I directed him to Stratford-on-Avon and suggested that he should fill in the rest of his time by visiting an English country house. He arrived the following afternoon, and I was a little anxious as to how he would react when we went down to the lake to bathe. I thought of telling everyone to wear a swimming-suit, but discarded the idea because it would have caused the children to regard him as an oddity.

He looked a little startled when the younger ones dropped their clothes on the bank and plunged into the water.... I had told them all to be properly dressed for tea. When the older ones did the same he ran back to the house . . . but only to fetch his cine-camera. He expended three reels of film as they dived from the branches of an oak tree, swam out to collect water lilies, raced through the meadows. "It is like Eden!" he exclaimed ecstatically. "What a wonderful lesson it will be for my congregation. I shall tell the narrow-minded members that it is *they* who are the serpents!"

Fortunately, as he told me in many letters, his congregation responded very warmly, and he showed his film so often that he had to have several new prints of it.

Even children who had been constantly told, "Don't touch . . . you'll get dirty!" or "Don't touch . . . you'll break it!" soon learned to feel an object instead of merely looking at it. With very little practice they could identify thirty or more species of leaves with their eyes shut, and became alive to the subtleties of texture possessed by many different kinds of wood and stone and fabric.

An interesting sidelight was that as they began to "see" with their hands they began to take much better care of them. Two confirmed nail-biters spontaneously cured themselves of this unattractive habit because they found it interfered with the pleasure of feeling with their fingertips. Their manual dexterity increased to a remarkable degree, and not only in such obvious ways as being able to knock in a nail without hitting their thumbs, or repairing their bicycles efficiently, but in the benign direction in which they employed their reawakened talents. Very soon I could trust any of them to take a tick from a dog's ear without leaving the head embedded, or to remove burrs from a girl's hair without making her wince . . . an expertise never achieved by any of my nannies. It was my daughter who taught me the best way of removing grit from an eye. A child had fallen flat on his face in the sand of the riverbank, and I was licking the corner of a handkerchief and twisting it into a point as a preliminary to removing the debris, when Gillian exclaimed, "Oh, Joan, don't be so silly. *Lick* it out! Your tongue is much softer than a handkerchief." Which of course it is, and also very much more effective.

Not long ago I recalled a happy and acceptable life as a Chinese concubine. From early childhood she was taught how to increase the flexibility of her hands and the sensitivity of her fingertips. By the time she was thirteen, the difference between the texture of one type of flower petal and another, and even the texture of different species of plums, was as obvious to her as the difference between linen and tweed would be to most people. To protect her fingertips when off duty she wore artificial nails, their length and the metal from which they were made being a symbol of her excellence in the art of love . . . just as the height of a chef's bonnet is a symbol of his place in the hierarchy of the artists in cooking. She lived a couple of thousand years ago; and as the Chinese also forgot that love, in all its aspects, is the greatest of the Arts, the original significance of the finger-guards was forgotten, and Chinese women grew non-retractable claws as a status symbol.

I believe that the cultivation of the senses is of vital importance because they must either develop or diminish: they cannot remain static. The senses can remain acute and fully effective even in extreme old age, but only in individuals who have put them to full use. Such annoyances as being "hard of hearing," or myopic, are not, as is often presumed, natural handicaps of the elderly; they are often the results of nothing more nor less than sensory laziness. If this laziness continues too long, then the supra-physical can become seriously depleted in this particular respect, and in a subsequent incarnation the individual may find himself in a body which reflects these deficiencies, and may even be born blind or deaf. There are, of course, other causes of these disabilities, but I am convinced that by far the most common one is a sense which has been neglected until it has atrophied.

Among the benefits which would accrue from a widespread cultivation of the senses would be a marked reduction in the deaths which are caused by the slow suffocation of boredom. The numbers self-doomed to die of this malady can be seen in every restaurant, in every resort, among every plod of tourists. Yet the sad state of the bored and boring is totally unnecessary at any age, for the truly perceptive are never dull, and pleasure not patience is their criterion of companionship.

There would also be a sharp drop in the incidence of sexual crime, and in the promiscuity which results from neither of the players having been able to suggest anything else to do. For when a body has lost the use of one of its senses, the energy deprived of its normal outlet will flow into the others, which is why the blind usually develop an increased acuity of hearing and touch. So if in successive incarnations an individual has made little use of his sensory awareness, due perhaps to conditioning in a puritanical environment, the supra-physical may have become so inept that instead of dividing its energies appropriately it allows the major portion of them to be concentrated into the genitals; this target being chosen because the reproductive urge has existed since our earliest animal incarnations and therefore is so deeply ingrained in our memories that it is the last instinct to be abandoned.

Because so many psychiatric patients were born still suffering from the consequences of the delusion that merit could be acquired by bullying their bodies, it is not surprising that a psychiatric theory which discounts reincarnation presumes that it is normal for infants to be obsessed with their sexual drive. But though such sad little savages are likely to arrive in increasing numbers unless the present generation adopts a more sane sensory ethic, they will still only be terrifying examples of how a personality can become crippled by false concepts as factually as a foetus can be crippled by thalidomide. The least we can do for our children is to try to ensure that they learn more closely to resemble the natural condition of man. Then the term "human nature" will no longer be used as an excuse for behaviour which is unnatural because it is very far from benign.

6

REINCARNATION
AND PSYCHOTHERAPY
by Denys Kelsey

I had always been appalled by the length of time an orthodox psychoanalysis was presumed to require; and one appeal of hypnosis had been that with its aid a radical form of therapy could be accomplished far more quickly. I completely accepted Joan's concept of the vastly increased time-scale during which the events responsible for a patient's illness might have occurred, and I found it extremely exciting. But I was apprehensive that the task of searching for the essential experience in this virtually limitless area might be endless.

Joan assured me that she was well aware that some patients would seize on the notion of reincarnation as a new avenue of escape, but she felt confident of being able to discriminate between a genuine recall from an earlier lifetime and an alleged memory which in fact was only a fantasy in fancy dress. She emphasised that in the majority of cases the cause of the neurosis would lie in events of the current lifetime, and that only when fragments of an earlier personality had failed to integrate would the proposed extension of my usual regression technique become apposite.

We had scarcely established ourselves in London when two such cases occurred in quick succession.

They were particularly impressive to me because each was a former patient on whom, long before I had even heard of Joan, I had carried out an extensive hypno-analysis which had been only partially successful.

The first was a young man with an obsessional neurosis. His most prominent symptom was the unshakeable idea that an action he had performed when a boy of seven was responsible for the arthritis which his father developed some thirteen years later.

The incident had happened when his parents, who had been away for a few days, were due to return, and his nanny had asked him to help her to make their bed. She had gone to fetch the sheets when it occurred to him to run a damp flannel over the mattress—a task he had completed before she reentered the room.

He knew that to associate this incident with his father's illness was completely illogical, but this in no way diminished his feelings of guilt and anxiety. And, as so frequently happens in this obsessional type of illness, the mechanism responsible for his principal symptom had spread to various other aspects of his emotional life and created a number of subsidiary problems.

The analysis went into many ramifications which it is unnecessary to consider here; but I must mention certain factors which concerned the central symptom. According to a theory which at that time I considered basic, every small boy goes through a phase of feeling violently hostile towards his father. If this hostility, instead of being resolved, is relegated to the child's unconscious, it may later be the source of a wide variety of neurotic feelings. I assumed that this was what had happened in this case. And when I learned, during an early session, it was axiomatic in his family that to sleep in a damp bed meant "catching your death of cold" or resulted in "rheumatism," I felt sure that in running a damp flannel over the mattress the child had been acting out an unconscious wish to kill his father.

I no longer believe that it is natural for small boys to go through this hostile phase, but this patient had undoubtedly done so. To his astonishment and dismay he found a plethora of such feelings and a number of acts through which they had found symbolical expression. But to my surprise, the damp flannel episode did not appear to come under this heading. Though I returned to the point repeatedly, and the patient appreciated how apt an explanation it would be, it had no effect on his obsession. After about eighty sessions it became clear that we were making no further progress, so we mutually agreed to discontinue the analysis.

I heard from him occasionally, so I knew that his symptoms waxed and waned but were not preventing him making excellent progress in his career. I had had no news of him for two years when a letter arrived asking for an appointment as soon as possible. He wrote that a few months previously his father had died of a stroke. This event had caused no exacerbation of my patient's symptoms until he had chanced upon an article in a magazine which mentioned that if rats were exposed for long enough to cold and damp they suffered a rise in blood pressure. This information had sparked off the chain of ideas: "Cold . . . damp . . . high blood pressure . . . stroke!" And now he felt that not only his father's arthritis but his death also was inexorably linked to the episode of the damp mattress.

When he arrived, I gave him a brief resumé of my reasons for believing that the origin of his symptom might lie in an earlier lifetime. He found the theory acceptable, and readily agreed that Joan should be present during the session.

Within minutes of reaching deep hypnosis, he said, "I can see a young woman in Edwardian dress . . . she is wearing a wide-brimmed hat tied on with a veil . . . she is standing on the steps outside the front-door, waiting to be taken out in the motor-car which she is hoping to see come up the drive leading to the house. . . it is a large mansion . . ."

At this point, Joan passed me the notebook by which she communicates with me during a session, as even a low whisper can be disturbing to the patient. I read, "Valid memory—I can see it too. But not a mansion—an ordinary late-Victorian house. Ask him, 'How many windows?' "

I did so. He replied, "There are two on each side of the front-door, which has four steps leading up to it . . . there are five windows in the upper story." Then he added, "I can see the drive clearly now . . . it is only a gravel sweep round a shrubbery of laurels."

During the next hour the story gradually unfolded. The young woman had been orphaned during her early teens when her parents died during a cholera epidemic in India. "My father was in the Army and my mother had always been delicate." She had been sent back to England to live with her aunt, her mother's elder sister. The house was on the outskirts of a country town which the patient thought was in East Anglia, but he could not remember the name of it. She imagined herself to be financially dependent on her aunt until recently, at the age of twenty-one, she had been told by a lawyer that her parents had left her a substantial trust fund. Until she married, the interest was controlled by the aunt, but on her marriage the capital would become her own: providing, and this was the crux of the problem, that the marriage took place with her aunt's consent. If she married someone considered "undesirable," she would not get a penny of it.

The patient became increasingly emotional as he described how the girl hoped to marry the curate, whom the aunt did not consider a "suitable match." Perhaps the curate was too timid or too avaricious to agree to an elopement, but it became obvious that the girl was becoming desperate with the fear of losing him.

At this stage, Joan handed me another note: "Tell him to see his aunt's bedroom."

He soon began to describe a room which was obviously the lair of a professional invalid. "It is intolerably stuffy: she has been burning one of her medicated cones and she never permits a window to be opened . . . there are medicine bottles and pill boxes everywhere."

Another note from Joan: "Ask what the aunt is doing."

The immediate response to this question was, "She is having a bath . . . it has mahogany sides and there is a step up to it . . ."

I asked him what he was doing. He replied, "I am making her bed while she is in the bath. But I do not get the sheets from the airing cupboard—I bring them from the clothesline in the garden."

At this point, Joan, unseen by the patient whose eyes remained closed while under hypnosis, made the gesture of dipping her hand in water and flicking the drops from her fingers. But before I could ask him for further details, he continued: "The sheets are damp . . .but not damp enough! I go to the washstand to fetch the ewer . . . and flick water over the mattress . . ."

But the aunt came back from the bathroom too soon. She not only saw what the girl was doing but understood why she was doing it. She screamed, "You want me to catch my death of cold!" and fell into such a frenzy of rage that she had a stroke. From this she remained bedridden for many years, nursed by the girl, who dared not leave her because the aunt now had the additional weapon of the threat to expose the attempt at murder.

When I brought the patient slowly back to the present day and out of hypnosis, he had a clear memory of all he had been telling us and felt no doubt at all that it was a part of his own long-history. He was completely satisfied that at last he had discovered the true source of his guilt—a guilt which had become transferred to his father. When I wrote to him for permission to quote from his case history, he confirmed that this symptom had never recurred after this session.

The second of these two cases arrived a few days later. The patient was a tall, wiry, athletic young man who suffered from the idea that there was something feminine about the shape of his hips. This idea was associated with feelings of guilt and inferiority so intense that he had been unable to concentrate on training for a career and was ill at ease with both men and women. The knowledge that both the idea and the feelings were completely irrational was of no help to him whatever.

He was an unusually good hypnotic subject, and I am satisfied that during the course of a long analysis I did not overlook any factor in his present life which might have been the origin of his symptoms. I managed to help him to the extent that he was able to derive considerable enjoyment from social activities, and also to complete an arduous training for a profession. But I knew that I had failed to solve his essential problem.

After we had discontinued the analysis he used to visit me perhaps once a year, but socially rather than professionally. I had not seen him for an unusually long time when he wrote asking for an appointment because his symptoms were again troubling him severely.

He was sympathetic to my new ideas and was obviously pleased that Joan was also going to try to help him. I induced hypnosis and told him to let his mind wander in search of the origin of his feelings, stressing that he would have no hesitation about expressing anything, even though it seemed improbable or bizarre.

Within a few minutes he began to describe scenes in which an elegant young woman appeared, always with a handsome escort. But the scenes changed abruptly: swathed in white ermine she was alighting from a Daimler at the entrance to the Savoy, and then, without any thread of continuity, she was on the deck of a large yacht and then in the paddock at Ascot.

Joan handed me a note. "This is a genuine recall. But he is not seeing the girl he really was: these are the girl's daydreams of the woman she longed to be. Tell him to see the girl herself."

He quickly identified with her, using the present tense and becoming increasingly distressed as the story progressed. She had been the daughter of a small tradesman in a university town, and had fallen in love with a titled undergraduate. She believed he intended to marry her, and her fantasies were of the life she expected to lead as his wife, a role for which she tried to equip herself by poring over fashion magazines and "society" papers.

But when she told him that she thought she might be pregnant, he was too scared even to be sympathetic and said he never wished to see her again. She resorted to purging, excessively hot baths, and to jumping from a five-foot wall: but none of these devices had the desired effect. She laced herself into a strong corset in anguished apprehension of the day when her remorselessly swelling abdomen must betray her condition to her parents. At five months, in desperation, she sought an abortion at unskilled hands.

Many of the grisly details were described. The operation took place in the kitchen of a squalid little house and was performed by an old woman who presumably panicked or fled in search of help when she realised that something had gone seriously wrong. The girl died still strapped down on the table: listening to her blood dripping on the stone floor, as she became increasingly cold, increasingly terrified.

It was the circumstances of this death, alone and in fear, which caused an element of her personality to become split off and frozen in a timeless present. The integrated components reincarnated within two years, but in a male body. Had this body been female, my patient might have suffered from an irrational fear of childbirth, or from phantom pregnancies. It is a tribute to his basic stability that although he was in effect being haunted by his own ghost, its appeal for integration was translated only as "a feeling that there is something feminine, something shameful, about the shape of my hips."

The other aspect of this case which to me was of special interest was that the fantasies which were seen both by the patient and by Joan during the initial phase of the session had appeared during the earlier hypnoanalysis. I had felt these scenes to be important and had urged him to enlarge upon them, but he had been unable to do so. I had offered various interpretations, including the possibility that the elegant woman represented the person he unconsciously wished to be. He could reply only that none of these interpretations felt valid, and there was no trace of the indignation which often indicates that a suggestion is correct but has been offered prematurely. In retrospect this is not surprising, since he, and I, were thinking in terms of only a single lifetime.

When discussing the case with Joan, I asked her how she had recognised that these fantasies, although highly relevant, were not memories of actual events. She explained that the clue lay in the fact that they were static and contained no action. This was because the girl was able to visualise how she would appear, but not what she would do, in situations which were outside her social experience. Had she belonged to the same milieu as the man she hoped to marry, she would have seen herself playing an active part in her daydreams, in which case their true nature would have been more difficult to discern.

The fantasies had persisted because the girl had directed such a large proportion of her energies into her hopes for the future, and then into her apprehensions of what would ensue if her pregnancy were discovered. It was this disproportionate quota of energy which had caused the fantasies to become condensed into constructs having an independent existence of their own, on the wish-fear level of reality. If they had been only ephemeral, they could not have been perceptible to anyone else.

Had I followed the thread of the fantasies which was offered to me during the hypno-analysis, I might have unravelled this patient's problem very much sooner. But I could not do so, because it led me beyond the limits of a single lifetime which then circumscribed my approach to psychiatry. But when I no longer tried to fit the relevant material into too small a framework, his symptoms, with Joan's help, were cured in a single session. I think the word "cured" is justified, for he has had no recurrence of symptoms during eight years, and he is very happily married.

The two cases which I have just described belong to the group of neuroses which are caused by fragments of the personality having become dissociated; the contribution of reincarnation is the recognition that such fragments sometimes derive from an earlier personality. But a far more common cause of neuroses is a defect in character. In cases of this type, the effect of reincarnation, perhaps surprisingly, has been to focus my attention less upon the patient's past than upon his present.

The key to this change of emphasis, although I then did not realise it, had been offered to me in the different reactions displayed by patients when regressed to interuterine life. For example, some reacted to sensations of discomfort by an aggressive desire to retaliate; others by trying to make themselves inconspicuous, in the hope of escaping from further attack. I had also noted that the patient's approach to life when adult was essentially similar to that which he had revealed while still a fœtus. But until I had widened the range of my concepts I did not realise the essential point: that an individual incarnates with the character he has acquired during the course of his long-history. And moreover that character is neither inherited nor moulded by the pressures of the environment, but is formed only by the exercise of the individual's power of choice. Outside pressures can cause a person to change his behaviour, but only he himself can change his intentions.

This principle is now the basis of my approach to the neurosis which is due to a character defect—an apparently fixed tendency to repeat a choice which is unhealthy—because I have become convinced that no matter how long a person may have had such a tendency, nor under what circumstances it was originally formed, he can begin to change it at any moment that he decides to do so.

The criterion as to whether a particular reaction is healthy or unhealthy derives from the undeniable fact that, with the possible exception of acute pain, the one situation which a human being finds intolerable is loneliness—the feeling that there is no one who is other than indifferent to the fact of his existence. And every action or reaction in respect of another person must either be heading away from loneliness or towards it, for it is to indifference that love will turn if it is not nourished, and to which even hate will eventually cool.

The effect of reincarnation is to underline the force of the word "eventually," for the end of a lifetime is not necessarily the end of a tendency to a particular type of reaction. The time must come when the approach of loneliness on account of unhealthy traits engenders a degree of anxiety which manifests itself as one or another of a wide variety of neurotic symptoms. But if the patient can be shown the aspects of his character which are threatening him with loneliness and can form the wholehearted wish to change them, then the change will begin and the symptoms will start to recede.

A question which I am often asked is whether every patient who is able to reach a deep state of hypnosis can be regressed to an earlier lifetime. In the majority of patients with whom, for one reason or another, I have used hypnosis, the need to explore an earlier lifetime has not arisen: and among those in whom I thought a previous personality might be relevant, only a small proportion have been able to recall a single episode. Even when a patient is intellectually convinced of the concept of reincarnation and only seeks empirical evidence of personal continuity I cannot always help him to gain it. For instance, I had a patient who was so eager to have a glimpse of some episode in her long-history so that she could speak about the concept with more authority, that she devoted twelve sessions to this project, although the problem for which she had originally consulted me had already been resolved.

I had had ample evidence that she was an excellent hypnotic subject, so when she said that her failure must be due to her inability to be hypnotised I told her to hold her left arm out at a right-angle and then suggested that she would forget about her arm until I told her to take it down. I brought her out of hypnosis, and Joan suggested that she might like to stay to tea. For an hour she sat, happily chatting, oblivious of the fact that her arm was still extended. Only when I told her to put it down did she realise what she had been doing: needless to say, I should not have performed this elementary experiment unless I had known that it would not cause her even momentary discomfort.

One might have thought that her eagerness for personal proof would have caused her imagination to produce some more or less convincing fantasy, especially as she had read all Joan's books and had felt, as we did, even at our first meeting, that we were old friends. Certainly she is a woman of outstanding integrity, but, contrary to my expectations, I have found that nearly every patient has shown this same determination not to fake.

Considering the prevalence of claims to far memory which to me seem obviously spurious, I find it interesting that even when a patient has recovered an episode which appears essentially plausible, although in fact it has become grossly distorted in transit to his present consciousness, it is often he who first questions its validity. It is widely held that patients tend to produce the type of material which will please their psychiatrist, but mine have seldom done so; presumably because their desire to be relieved of their symptoms was more important to them than the time-wasting ploy of trying to lead their therapist astray.

It is also probable that Joan's presence at a session acts as a deterrent to patients who might otherwise employ their imaginations in an attempt to delude or impress. Although there are occasions, for instance if she is in pain or very tired, when her faculties are temporarily inactive, under normal conditions she can tune in to the episode which the patient is reliving, especially if the episode concerns a split-off fragment of one of his earlier personalities. She explained to me that the reason she finds it so easy to share the patient's identification with his "ghost" is not merely that she has had considerable experience of coping with this type of phenomenon, but because a ghost, by its very nature, has so often repeated the circumstances in which its energy is bound that the emotion is deeply etched, the situation clearly delineated, the background specific.

I have found that it is very unusual for a patient to remember the name he bore in an earlier lifetime, or to be able to date an episode which he has been able to relive in most graphic detail. This may be due to the fact that the incidents which my patients have recalled under hypnosis were directly concerned with the origin of their symptoms, and therefore are not memories which stemmed from integrated components of their personalities but from the ghosts which had become split off by some traumatic event.

A ghost exists in a circumscribed present which contains emotions and sensations but no knowledge of matters which are primarily intellectual. For instance, the girl dying of hemorrhage would have thought of herself as "I" and not by name, and the date of the abortion would not have been associated with her pain and terror. Joan was able to date this girl's death, and therefore to know that there was an interval of less than two years before she incarnated in a male body, only because the clothes which played such an important part in her fantasies were in the fashion of 1927, a fact which Joan happened to remember because it was the year she bought her trousseau.

One of the few occasions when a patient produced a date which was of intrinsic interest occurred in 1959. I can best describe him as a stalwart yeoman. Following an accident in which he wrenched his shoulder very severely, he had developed a disability in his right hand which was clearly not due to any organic cause. He was referred to me in the hope that hypnotherapy might help where a more orthodox psychiatric approach had failed. Except for his disability he was in excellent physical health and, mentally, an exceptionally well-balanced man. He had left school at the age of thirteen, so as to be able to contribute to the support of his family, and so far as I was able to discover his historical knowledge was virtually non-existent. His recreations were gardening, carpentry, and swimming: he seldom went to the cinema: had neither a radio nor a television, and was not interested in books.

He entered hypnosis very easily, and he had been

recounting some episode from his boyhood when he paused and then said, "I am seventeen, and I am very ill. But not so ill as some of the other sailors."

As his current history had contained no mention of a severe illness or that he had ever been to sea, I asked, "When did this happen?" He replied, without hesitation, "In 1567."

While I was still assimilating the fact that my patient was now in the reign of Elizabeth the First instead of Elizabeth the Second, he proceeded to describe his symptoms: the bleeding gums and loosening teeth, the stinking breath, the bruises which appeared without any blow to cause them, and the increasing weakness. He described, in fact, a typical case of scurvy.

After he had recounted many vivid scenes of his experiences while an Elizabethan seaman, I asked him whether his ship had fought against the Armada. He seemed puzzled, and then replied, "I do not know what you mean by the Armada." But when during the next session, I asked, "When did you die?" he answered, "In 1593. Five years after we sank the accursed Spaniards."

My memory for dates is exceedingly hazy, so I had to wait until I got home to confirm that the Spanish Armada was defeated in 1588, five years prior to the date he had given for his own death. The reason he was puzzled when I first asked him about the Armada was, I feel sure, that he was regressed then to a period of his Elizabethan life which antedated this event by several years. Obviously he could not remember a sea battle which, from that point of view, had not yet happened.

When a patient is assisted by hypnosis to release the energy which has become trapped in a fragment of a previous personality, he may either have an intense abreaction, or else, whilst still attaining a therapeutic degree of identification, he may remain sufficiently detached to be both spectator and participant of the crucial event. I am not able to predict with any confidence which of these two courses a patient is likely to

141

follow, nor if he encounters more than one ghost during his treatment that his reaction will be consistent. I presume therefore that the immediate impact of a recall depends on the energy-content of the ghost and not on the qualities of the present personality.

The recall of an event which occurred centuries ago can be as vivid as the memory of an automobile accident which occurred last week. In fact more vivid, for one is insulated by the intervening clock-time from a memory in normal-waking-consciousness, but a regression can have a sense of immediacy which is enveloping and absolute.

I gained empirical evidence of the intensity of such a recall on the first occasion that I relived an episode from my own long-history. I was very doubtful of being able to recover anything, especially as hypnotists are notoriously difficult to hypnotise, and Joan has no expertise in this particular technique. I advised her to follow the procedure which she had seen me use with patients; but instead she lit a candle and told me to stare at the flame. She averred that this was a method of inducing a level-shift that had once been a commonplace to us both and which I might again find effective.

Although rather nettled that she was ignoring my advice, I fixed my gaze on the flame and gave myself suggestions of relaxation.

The transition of a sceptical psychiatrist lying on his own couch to a man racing a chariot was instantaneous. On my left there was a barrier surrounding an island of spectators in the centre of the arena. On my right a chariot was overtaking me. I knew I should give way to it, but instead I forced my pair into the narrowing gap. There was a shuddering impact as our wheels interlocked. I was catapulted forwards and felt a wheel run over my chest. As the chariot overturned, it swung the horses against the barrier. The last thing I remembered was their screaming.

At this point, Joan brought me back to the present. But the terrible realisation that through a desire to show off I had caused the destruction of a pair of beloved horses brought a degree of shame which in my current life I had never previously experienced. There was no possibility of dissociating myself from this event: that it had occurred two thousand years ago was entirely irrelevant. It was I who had done it; and it was happening now. For forty-eight hours I felt I would never be able to face myself again.

Some months later, the thread of my debt to horses reappeared when Joan, for other reasons entirely, was recalling episodes from a life we had shared, also as husband and wife, in England at the end of the eighteenth century. Among the many details which emerged was that my life centred round horses. I bred them and schooled them, and sometimes gave one to a trusted friend. But I never sold any, which is probably why our house became increasingly dilapidated. So anxious was I never to cause them discomfort, that I forbade steel to be put in their mouths and always rode them on a bit made of leather.

My attempt to redress the equine balance must have persisted into my present life. Riding was my favourite hobby, and a horse I schooled during my period in the Army only just missed being selected for a British Olympic show jumping team. But though I enjoyed show jumping, hunting, and the occasional point-to-point, I was a poor competitor because I could never bring myself to take an avoidable risk of injuring the horse. Joan, of course, knew of my interest in horses; but what she did not know, because it had never occurred to me to tell her, was that I found the idea of putting steel in their mouths so distasteful, that whenever possible I used a bit made of rubber.

The incident of recalling a fragment of my own long-history was soon followed by my first experience of handling an episode from a patient's earlier life without Joan's help. At this period, she was not working with me as a routine because she was finishing a book which had been commissioned before our meeting.

The patient was a highly cultured professional man in his mid-forties, who since puberty had been exclusively homosexual. In retrospect it is surprising that in a case of this nature I did not moot the possibility of reincarnation at an early stage, but there are two reasons why I did not do so. First, as I cannot emphasise too often or too strongly, recognition that the current life is but the most recent of many is by no means a panacea. In the majority of cases the root of a neurosis lies in the present, can be found in the present, and can be resolved in the present. Therefore, except in unusual instances, it would be foolish to omit a scrutiny of the patient's existing circumstances; and to understand these fully, a consideration of his childhood is sometimes unavoidable.

Second, during our initial interview, this patient had declared that he was a staunch upholder of orthodox Church of England doctrine, and from this I inferred that he might find the idea of reincarnation unacceptable. Success in therapy seldom depends upon a patient sharing this belief, and many treatments run their course without the concept being mentioned; but needless conflict, evoked by introducing this highly controversial issue when it is not necessary, can delay rather than accelerate the process.

So the first thirteen sessions were devoted to exploring his present life, both with and without the aid of hypnosis. But I found nothing of sufficient emotional significance to account for the compulsive drive which caused him to seek a male companion as the only way of assuaging his loneliness. This loneliness was the core of his problem; for however long and arduously he tried to cure himself by being ascetic, his self-imposed solitude eventually became intolerable. Then he would enter into yet another of the relationships which, as he expressed it, "seemed foredoomed to failure and to leave me lonelier than ever."

At the fourteenth session he arrived in a state of acute agitation, due to the fact that since we last met he had moved into a new apartment; and within two days had found himself strongly attracted to a young man living in the same building.

I induced hypnosis, with the intention of telling him to try to pinpoint what aspect of this particular young man made him seem so desirable. But instead, I found myself saying, "See *who* is causing you to have these feelings."

Within seconds, he had begun to describe episodes from a life in which he had been "the Hittite wife of the governor of the foreigners who have invaded my country." The marriage was at first exceedingly satisfactory, for she lived in unaccustomed luxury, and was fawned upon by sycophants who knew that her husband often turned to her for advice. Then he received orders which would entail his absence from his headquarters for some considerable time, and by overruling his objections, she was able to accompany him.

By questions concerning the direction of the march, the character of the terrain, and the number of days which elapsed between the various periods when "The army went into temporary encampment," I tried to gain information about the scope and aims of this campaign. Perhaps if my patient had been recalling his experiences as a soldier, he would have retained this kind of data, but the woman he had been remembered only the discomforts she had suffered on this seemingly interminable journey; the aches and fevers, the heat and the boredom, the dust-storms and the sand flies.

When I asked, "How long did the journey last?" the reply was, "Far, far longer than I had anticipated. The hardships which I was forced to endure destroyed my health and my beauty. And then my husband came no more to my tent to visit me."

When she reached home, her bitterness increased. Her husband no longer asked her advice, nor did he bother to conceal that neither her thoughts nor her body aroused his interest. Already acutely jealous, she became obsessed with hatred when she discovered that she had been supplanted not by another woman, but by a handsome boy.

This final humiliation caused her to steal her husband's dagger so that it could become the object on which to focus the energy of a curse.

"I took it to a Priest of Baal, and paid him much gold to curse the owner of the dagger: 'May everything he finds sweet become bitter. May everyone he lives for, die.'"

I asked, 'When did you die?"

He cried out, "I was soon murdered...I was stabbed!"

As he was obviously in considerable emotional distress, I brought him back to the present and out of hypnosis. He retained a clear memory of everything he had recounted, and I asked him to give an opinion of the woman's character.

He exclaimed, "She was a terrible creature! She did not love her husband, even at the beginning; she only coveted the prestige that marriage to him would bring. She did not go with him on his journey because she wanted to share its hardships: she went only to prove to him that he could not do without her: that although a woman, she was stronger even than he. Her jealousy was wicked enough: but to inflict a curse upon him was an unforgiveable sin."

Knowing that he was truly devout, I said to him, "Imagine that you are a priest. Imagine that a woman has confessed this story to you. She understands the nature and the magnitude of her transgressions, and has resolved never to act in this way again. What would you say to this woman?"

146

He replied without hesitation, "I would give her Absolution."

So I asked him to absolve the woman who was part of his total self.

He knelt in prayer. Of the form of his prayers I know nothing; but even from my chair on the other side of the room I could feel the beneficent energy which was flowing from him. At length he rose to his feet; and I saw that the drawn, anxious expression on his face with which I had become so familiar had changed to a serene contentment. He said, "I know it is finished. I am no longer a homosexual."

He came to see me some weeks later, but only to confirm that he was free, and knew he would remain so.

Then I did not hear from him for four years. His letter contained the sentence, "The cure, by the way, through far-memory, and what I can only regard as your exorcism, has been effective indeed; and I have found myself able to enter a wholly satisfactory hetero-sexual relationship."

7

THE AGE OF PERCEPTION
by Joan Grant

The first time I noticed how clearly the newborn reveal their essential character, even to the amateur eye, was on the 22nd April 1952: the day Gillian had her first baby.

The private rooms of the hospital opened on a wide corridor, in which the infants were parked in cots outside their mothers' doorways except at feeding times. Inspired by grandmotherly interest, I inspected a row of about a dozen. The first three or four, who were all over a week old, had a surprisingly wide range of physical appearance yet still looked just like babies. The next one, born during that night, was an exceedingly malevolent man, glaring at me from an infant body; so malevolent that I felt it would be a service to humanity to throw him out of the window. However had anyone done so he would have foisted himself on some other unfortunate couple, if not on the same parents, within the minimum period.

I happened to mention this incident when lecturing in New York, and afterwards had expert confirmation from a member of the audience. She was the sister in charge of the obstetrics theatre of a large hospital, a post she had held for over twenty years. Even during her midwifery training she had noticed that the infant reveals its basic characteristics immediately after birth, although after a few hours these cease to be so clearly discernible until several weeks or even months later. She told me that she had found it difficult to conceal from mothers who had produced exceedingly unpleasant individuals that she knew they deserved condolences rather than congratulations.

She had made detailed notes of every baby whom she had thought would be outstanding in any particular direction, and kept in touch with the mothers so that she could check her observations. She had proved correct in such a very high percentage of cases that it could not be dismissed as coincidence. Her empirical conviction that the character of an infant is formed long before it is born, and has a range which cannot be accounted for by intrauterine experience, had caused her to have complete certainty of the validity of reincarnation.

The reason why it is easier to assess the character at birth than during the subsequent weeks is that the ordeal mobilises aspects of the personality which will scarcely be in evidence again until the infant's field of choice begins to broaden. But should the body be in danger, these aspects may be remobilised: it is not only dehydration which sometimes causes a baby who is ill to look so old and wise.

The ability of this talented theatre sister to judge the basic characteristics of the newborn would have been put to full use in a more enlightened culture. For instance, in early dynastic Egypt she would have been one of the experts who, whenever possible, were present at a birth, so that the parents could be advised as to which aspects of their child's personality should be encouraged to flourish, and which aspects they should help him to change. For it was then recognised that the earlier he began to change his unhealthy attributes the easier it would be for him to do so.

Nowadays, any curative procedure directed at trying to help a baby, or even a small child, to change his ominous attitudes is usually foiled by the protest, "But he is only a baby! He is too *young* to understand!"

The real nexus of the problem is that unless he is taught how to redirect his energies while the acute perception of infancy is still relatively unobscured by brain function, his reeducation will be far more difficult, both for himself and everyone in his environment, than it need have been.

My ability to recall episodes from my current life's infancy without the aid of hypnosis is not a side-effect of the far-memory faculty, and I am sure that similar recalls could be done by almost anyone. But any form of recall requires the genuine wish to accept full responsibility for the experience, and will not occur when the motive is a search for some convenient scapegoat.

It is always painful to remember the virtues one has discarded, the abilities one has failed to employ, the insight one has failed to use; yet this can be very salutary, for it reminds one that all these attributes which one had when an infant, can, if one chooses, be rescued. I believe the reason so few patients produce therapeutic recalls during orthodox analysis is because they have been led to expect to find that as infants they were a horrid bundle of anti-social feelings, orientated towards scatology, patricide, mum-rape and sibling slaughter. Fortunately, in the vast majority of cases, such fantasies are born only in the minds of their analysts.

I am going to recount a few episodes from my early childhood because I think they are typical of most children, and illustrate the normal child's powers of observation, his ability to work out a plan and carry it into effect, and the insight which allows him to see slap through the pretences with which grown-ups contrive to conceal themselves from each other. I think that if the perspicacity of the so-called Innocents were more widely recognised they would be taught how to use this perspicacity to good advantage; and they would also be unable to misuse it to make fools of their unfortunate parents.

The earliest decision I can remember making was when I refused to suckle, although I was by then becoming exceedingly thirsty because I had already several times rejected my mother's breast. The smell of her milk was nauseating; the reason for this instinctive reaction probably being that in it I could smell the drugs from which I had suffered during the foetal period, drugs which she took to combat severe attacks of asthma. I remember acute despair when I was offered a bottle only to find that it contained the same repugnant fluid . . . by this time I had a raging thirst and craved for water. I also remember the tremendous relief I felt when I was offered a bottle which contained a formula, which, years later, I identified, by the smell, as "Mellins Food."

I think it extremely probable that many of the infants who refuse to suckle have the same instinctive recognition that the mother's milk contains some constituent which has either caused them discomfort, or been actively dangerous to them, during their foetal period. So as there is an increasing tendency for pregnant women to be given tranquillisers, and other drugs whose effect on the unborn child is not fully understood, it is exceedingly important that the infant's natural desire to protect itself from an additional dose of something which has already proved unsatisfactory should be recognised and accepted. If an alternative form of nourishment is withheld, its protective mechanism will become numbed by hunger: or rather numbed by thirst, for again personal memory suggests that thirst, especially after prolonged crying, is far more insistent than hunger.

During my first four months I had the good fortune

151

to be looked after by an old-fashioned maternity nurse with whom it was very easy to communicate. She at once recognised the noise I made to indicate I wished to unload, and so provided a pot, tapping it with her finger to draw my attention to its convenient presence. Perhaps she learned this helpful technique through having handled many infants and so knew that it is much easier to house train them during their first weeks than it will be when they are older. Or she may have acquired this item of insight when belonging to a tribe who carry their infants on their backs. Such a mother, as I know from personal experience, takes the trouble to remain alert to signals from her infant, otherwise she will suffer the discomfort of hot trickles down her spine. Whatever the source of her expertise may have been, I benefitted from it exceedingly; for instead of having to endure the misery of soaking diapers I never had to wear one after the age of six weeks.

My mother, who very properly considered that every infant should have received similar servicing, used to infuriate parents of my generation by saying, "But your baby has *wet* itself! How *very* extraordinary. To look at it one would not have guessed that it was mentally deficient."

I tried to explain to her that modern theories of baby care maintained that terrible traumata were caused by early pot training. To which she briskly replied, "Well if the parents are silly enough to believe anything so idiotic I suppose one can only tell them that they should have been prevented from breeding."

When the maternity nurse left she was replaced by a nanny, and on the day she arrived I was taken to a furnished house which my parents had rented for the month of August 1907 . . . I having been born in that same year on the 12th April. Hoping to make the changeover easier, my mother decided to give me my bottle; which I indignantly rejected because it resonated me to being offered her breast. One must remember that in those days parents seldom handled their offspring, and would no more have thought of bathing their baby than of doing the washing-up, or of feeding it than of flustering the cook by invading her kitchen.

Not only had I been suddenly bereft of the only person with whom I could communicate, but all bottles were now suspect, for they had again become associated with the initial ones which had contained mother's milk. So the only course open to me was to refuse to accept anything unless it was offered in a spoon: spoons had proved safe, as they contained water when I was thirsty.

As I became increasingly hungry I thought of a spoon with growing desperation: its shape and colour and the feel of it touching my mouth. I beamed SPOON at everyone who came near me, and their failure to understand scared me, for it was very alarming to be at the mercy of bland giants who seemed so utterly stupid. I was at the point of allowing myself to be poisoned when a visitor suddenly understood what I was trying to convey. She told them to feed me with a spoon; and never before or since has a meal been quite so delectable.

I was able to check the date of this incident, and the accuracy of my visual observations, because I happened to mention to my father, some twelve years later, that I could remember a few events which had occurred before I was six months old. He asserted that this was impossible because my brain would have not yet been sufficiently developed. So I described the room which had been my nursery in considerable detail: the relative positions of the door, windows, and fireplace, and a semi-circular corner turret. I also recalled the colour and pattern of the wallpaper. I knew that the nursery was the second door on the left at the top of the front staircase, and that there was a window with blue, red, and yellow panes on the landing.

Fortunately Mother remembered that I had gone on a hunger strike when I was four months old, and also that it had taken place in the house we had occupied only during that August and to which none of us had been before or since.

My father, impelled by a spirit of scientific interest, took the trouble to go to the house to check my assertions. The new owners were delighted to let him see over it, but must have been rather startled when he asked their permission to strip off a piece of wallpaper from the recently redecorated room, the second on the left at the top of the front stairs, opening from a landing which was lit by a stained glass window. Under the new paper he found another, but this bore no resemblance to the one I had described. However he persisted with his investigations, and the next layer of paper was identical with the one he hoped, or feared, to find.

The wallpaper is relevant in another context: even at four months old I considered it painfully ugly. I used to stare at it in disgust; wishing my cot was closer to the window so that I could watch leaves moving or the shape of branches against the sky. I used to wonder why the walls of a room had such an uneasy pattern, such harsh colours, and such a horrid texture . . . for I could touch it by stretching my hand between the bars of my cot.

If it were recognised that the artistic sensibilities of infants have already been cultivated during many earlier lifetimes, parents would take the trouble not to assault them with needless ugliness. The attribute of "natural good taste" is inborn in most people, but often deliberately discarded during early childhood because having an "eye for beauty" entails the ability also to recognise the forms and colours which evoke pain instead of pleasure. If a child's surroundings are too inharmonious, if he sees too many grotesques in his picture books, he may either become purblind or even go one step further in the wrong direction and develop a perverted taste for forms and colours which his infant observation would instantly have recognised as being distorted.

I am not suggesting that the arrival of an infant involves the additional expense of employing an expert interior decorator. But I am suggesting that he should be given something beautiful to look at, and that this object should be changed sufficiently often to hold his attention. A single flower comfortably within eye range is an excellent way of providing him with hours of entertainment—but do not cheat him with a plastic flower, however satisfying these may be to adults. Choose his picture books with care: take the trouble to make a mobile of real things, leaves, shells, dried flowers, for him to watch. Put a branch of a pleasing shape where it can throw a pattern against a white wall—and do this when he is so young that the less discerning will say, with invincible stupidity, "But he is far too young to *notice!*" Such people will probably give him hideous toys whose only appropriate destination is the dustbin.

You will be amply rewarded for your efforts, even if you may suffer such momentary embarrassment as I suffered when Gillian, aged three, paused on the threshold of a banqueting hall which had been monstrously redecorated by a Victorian grandmother, and exclaimed to her hostess, "Oh who has been so cruel to this poor room!"

It is important to keep in mind that before a baby has learned to talk he will rely on telepathy, the method of communication common to all levels of experience except the three-dimensional. Suddenly to find oneself among people who cannot understand what one is trying to convey is exceedingly frustrating, as anyone knows who has found himself among foreigners whose language he cannot speak. In such a situation even adults are likely to shout, as though by sheer weight of decibels the word barrier could be shattered, and it is this same source of frustration which often causes babies to scream.

I recently came across a photograph of myself in the arms of an anxious father, at the age of ten months; and the sight of it brought a flashback to it being taken. The cumbersome box-camera, on a tripod, was draped with a black velvet pall, the lens covered with a leather cap, which was whisked off for the exposure. The photographer frequently popped his head under the pall and then bobbed out again, a performance which I found entertaining. Then he pointed to the lens-cover and said, in the cosy coo so repellent to children, "Watch for the little birdy to peep out! Tweet, tweet. Can't you hear it?"

I was hotly indignant that he could imagine I was silly enough to believe there was a bird in the box.

"Watch for the birdy! Tweet, tweet!" cajoled the photographer.

I tried to tell him not to be impertinent! How dared he insult my intelligence ... how dared he think I was a *baby!*

But I had no words, so I screamed with fury, and then wept because I was so helpless. The final humiliation came when my father said, "How extraordinary that the child should be frightened by a camera."

The loneliness of being unable to communicate through lack of language is one of the reasons why it is so reassuring to a baby to have an animal for a companion, for animals are also free from the limitations of speech. But the animal should be carefully chosen for its character; if it is basically jealous, bad-tempered, or aggressive the baby will recognise these traits more clearly than the average adult. The small child's longing for an animal is dimly recognised in the custom of providing him with stuffed toys. Perhaps a teddybear is better than nothing; but while a real animal increases his capacity for identification with another living being, with whom he can have an ambivalent current of affection and understanding, the teddy-bear is only an object on which he can project his fantasies, animate only in imagination. Imagination is a valuable asset, but only when it is used to supplement and correlate actual experience; it can be exceedingly dangerous when used as a substitute for reality.

I longed for an animal when I was a baby, but was considered too young to have one of my own: later experience suggests that nine months would have been the appropriate time, the age at which Gillian and a bull terrier puppy became mutually devoted companions.

The first animals whom I had the opportunity of knowing were two young chimpanzees, through the good fortune of having a nanny who was in love with the keeper who was training them. As we were then living in my grandmother's house on Primrose Hill, within easy pram-push of the Zoological Gardens, we visited them twice daily, while Mother imagined I was being aired in Regent's Park.

I was then about a year old, and it was exceedingly restful to have companions who also did not rely on speech. I had only to think "I would like a grape," for one of the chimpanzees carefully to select one from a box of sawdust and pop it into my mouth. They accepted me as easily as I accepted them. They carefully combed my hair with their fingers and I helped them to tie on their bibs, before the three of us sat amicably round a table and drank milk out of blue and white enamel mugs.

Children are capable of relating cause and effect at a much earlier age than is usually recognised. If their initiative is ignored, and the praise or scolding which they considered well earned fails to materialise, they may be extremely disquieted. Either their opinion of the grown-ups still further deteriorates, for it is impossible to rely on people who can be easily duped; or else the child considers his efforts so inconspicuous that this may lead to a feeling of unreality, which, if too often repeated, can contribute to a neurosis.

I was still about a year old when I heard my mother telling my half-sister Iris about the fire alarm which had been installed beside my parents' bed. She explained how it worked, and then added that it must never be used unless the fire was too serious to be coped with by the fire extinguishers: but it could summon fire engines which would arrive within minutes.

Even while I was listening to their conversation I made up my mind to summon fire engines at the earliest opportunity. I would have to be alone in my parents' bedroom; be able to climb on the bed without assistance; discover how to break the glass cover and then pull the brass knob. I understood perfectly well that this would be considered exceedingly naughty. At best I should be scolded, and at worst have my knickers removed and be put on a high marble-topped chest-of-drawers, a form of punishment known as "Putting-a-hot-baby-on-cold-marble," which I found intensely humiliating. It also scared me, because I was fearful of pitching off it onto my head. I knew I had died from falling from a height on some earlier occasion.

After a week of diligent practice I could climb onto even the highest bed. On the following day, I managed to escape from the nursery, when the gate at the head of the stairs was unlatched, and get undetected into my parents' bedroom. I could not reach the glass cover of the fire alarm until I had gained added height by standing on books which I piled on the bedside table, and was unable to break it until I realised that a soda water bottle which happened to be handy would make an excellent club. The knob was the next problem, but after tugging at it with mounting frustration I slipped off my vantage point, still clinging to the knob, and my weight dragged it out of its socket.

By the time the fire engines came clanging up the hill I was standing on a chair with my nose pressed against the windowpane. Firemen came running up the front steps, more firemen started unrolling a hose and unhooking ladders. Then I heard Father's voice assuring them that none of this was necessary as there was no fire . . . and more voices raised and expostulating. This was my moment of triumph, and I hurried downstairs, expecting to be praised first if punished later. I pointed at the largest fireman and then to myself shouting, "Me! Me! . . ." almost the full range of my vocabulary. The louder I shouted the louder I was shushed, until boiling with indignation at being ignored, I was carried off to the nursery.

Unless children's innate sense of justice has been blurred by brainwashing which has induced groundless guilt feelings, they can appear more ruthless than the average adult. When I was about four, the nanny I loved went for her summer holiday and was replaced by a "temporary" whom I detested. My cousin Westray, who was six and very strong for his age—he grew to be six foot eight—shared my opinion of her. Not only did she dislike us both but she was horribly cruel to mice. She set mousetraps in every cupboard, not spring traps which would at least have killed them quickly, but wire cages into which they were lured with cheese, only to be slowly drowned in the basin, while the fiend gloated over their dying struggles.

We did our best to avenge the mice by making the fiend's life as difficult as we could: but she was too large, too strong, too sly for us to do so effectively. She also constantly sneaked on us to our parents which led to further recriminations, and they refused to recognise her fiendishness because she had something incomprehensible called "Splendid References."

She had made me stand in the corner, and when this failed to do more than make me chant, "I love being in the corner because I can't see Nanny's horrid face," she pulled my hair so viciously that a strand of it came out in her hand. I had not noticed that Westray, always a loyal ally, was sitting on the floor taking off one of his new and heavy football boots. The fiend was glaring at me, red in the face and panting. I knew she was about to shake me till my teeth chattered. Westray stood up, the boot in his hand, and took careful aim. The boot hit her on the temple and she crumpled; and then fell flat on her back.

"I have killed her," said Westray, with calm satisfaction.

"And a very good thing too," I replied warmly.

"There will be a tremendous row," said Westray. "We shall be sent to bed without supper for at least a week."

"But well worth it. Think of the mice she drowned . . . she did not really deserve such a nice death." Then I added hastily, in case Westray should think I did not appreciate his splendid effort, "But we couldn't have drowned her. She is too big."

Not one twinge of remorse did either of us feel. A dead mouse more than cancelled out a dead fiend . . . and the fiend had killed enough mice to deserve a dozen executions.

At that moment Mother came into the room and exclaimed, "Is she drunk or has she fainted?"

I was about to say, "She is dead," wondering whether it was necessary to add that we had killed her, when to my dismay the fiend opened her eyes.

She failed to notice Mother, and glared with such ferocity at Westray that Mother said briskly, "Lie down at once: you are having a fit! How monstrous to take a post with children when you knew that you are an epileptic!"

I felt almost sorry for the fiend at that moment; for the more she tried to explain that she had been attacked by Westray the more firmly Mother became convinced that she was not only an epileptic but suffered from delusions which proved she was raving mad. Westray and I were sent out of the room and never saw the fiend again; for she had made the fatal mistake of being rude to Mother and so was sacked without notice.

Everyone was especially nice to us that day, to console us for the "terrible shock to our nerves," which we considered blissfully funny. After Westray had left I told Father what had really happened. He cautioned me, as I knew he would, not to mention the matter to Mother: and then laughed until laughter-tears made him have to polish his spectacles.

I received no religious education, and no one I had met ever went to church, but I presumed that even the most dim-witted adults knew that between bodies they went to the place I privately called the Beautiful Country. I had even temporarily held the theory that I could return there if I walked very slowly into the sea at low tide and went on walking until my hat floated off. I tried this on two occasions, at dawn before Nanny was awake, but funked going any further when the sea was up to my chin.

So when I suddenly realised that the man who was sitting opposite me at luncheon was going to die that night, it seemed natural to congratulate him on the fact that tomorrow would be his happiest birthday. He was a doctor of whom I was fond, so I was sad that I might not see him for some time, but knew that such feelings were exceedingly selfish. "It is not my birthday tomorrow," he said kindly. So I hastened to explain that I meant the kind of birthday that happened on the day one died.

I was dismissed from the dining room, soon to be followed by Mother, who scolded me severely for making such a cruel remark. Protests that it was not in the least cruel to congratulate someone I loved because something especially nice was about to happen to him were brushed angrily aside. I was at last reduced to tears, which though taken for tears of contrition were really of fury, at the total incomprehensibility of grown-ups, and was made to promise "never again to try to draw attention to myself by telling such wicked lies."

At last Mother calmed down sufficiently to say that I was unlikely to have done any harm, for the doctor was only fifty-five and knew he was perfectly healthy. But the row flared up again the following morning; when the doctor's body was found peacefully dead in its bed.

These two episodes, I think, well illustrate the attitude of normal children towards death. Their innate knowledge tells them that death is a trivial incident which they have often experienced, so they have no fear of it unless fear has been induced through stories of a vengeful god, eager to punish any behaviour considered "wicked" by the grown-ups, or descriptions of hell, or through hearing the dead talked about as though they were in dire need of sympathy. A slap-up funeral, especially viewing a corpse which has been turned by embalmers into a dreadful puppet, can cause even a robust child to have nightmares, which is yet another reason for condemning the current mortuary rites.

Death to healthy children means "to go somewhere else," so what is more natural than that they should wish that an irksome member of the household, who has refused to take hints that his absence would be a welcome relief, should depart by dying?

The view held by most psychoanalysts, that baby boys, at the drop of a diaper, would slay Pa so as to have a pop at Mum, is, I am convinced, nonsensical. But as many children have parents who cordially dislike each other, which the children know only too well even if parental rows never take place in their presence, they wish that one of the contestants would leave the arena so that there could be a bit of peace. Freud grew up in an environment where there was not only one Father figure making a nuisance of himself, but two generations of patriarchs living in the same house, so he would have had to be totally unrealistic not to have cordially wished them out of the way. But to him the patriarchs were invulnerable, even in fantasy, because behind them was Jehovah, an implacable God who demanded even such improbable sacrifices from male infants as their foreskins. So a perfectly healthy longing to be fledged was banished to Freud's unconscious until it emerged to be labelled the "Oedipus Complex."

A child who allows his perception to fall into disuse may gain short-term advantages: if he is clever enough to cozen his blood-kin he may become the focus of their anxieties, and if he has sufficient innate hatred he may feel strong through being a rebel. But he will buy this transient stability at a price which may impoverish his personality.

For not having retained the moral courage to see either himself or other people as they really are— which might be better or worse than he prefers to imagine he is only able to identify his fellow human beings by their status symbols, which seldom echo the quality of their hearts. Unless he regains his perception, his acquaintances may be numerous and his loins prolific; but he will always be lonely. For the man who is a stranger to himself lives among strangers.

His condition would be sad enough even if there were no natural gaps in temporal continuity: but we all wake in order to learn what we should do when we sleep; we are all born in order to acquire the compassion for which we shall be welcomed by our forerunners. To earn this welcome we have very often died, only to find that death dissipates our most cravenly cherished delusions.

Because we fear to be naked and unashamed, we scuttle back in search of another garment of flesh. But eventually we shall love enough, and be sufficiently loveable, to accept who we were, and are, and will be: for fig leaves are worn only by exiles from Eden.

8

PARENTHOOD
by Denys Kelsey

i. Would you really like a baby?
ii. Would a baby really like you?

The effects which parents may have upon their children have been the subject of endless consideration. But there is an aspect of parenthood which has tended to be neglected: the effects which a child may have upon its parents.

Adoption societies are so well aware of the stresses which a child will impose that they subject prospective foster-parents to a prolonged and detailed investigation. This will begin with enquiries into their financial circumstances and prospects, the accommodation they have to offer, and every aspect of their environment, and will extend to their religion, their work, their interests, and their habits.

Information will be required not only about their present state of health, but also about the medical history of themselves and their families. Is there any familial tendency, for instance, to cancer or heart trouble, or to any other condition suggesting a reduced expectation of life? On this question the nature of their favourite recreation may have an obvious bearing.

Then will come an expert assessment of the psychological state of the couple. In arriving at this, the adoption society will go into the mental history of the family of each of them, as well as the mental history of the couple themselves. And they will not merely want to find that there were no frank nervous breakdowns, but that there is positive evidence of stability in their records of performance both at school and at work.

They will be deeply interested in the strength of the relationship between the couple, and will listen with a particularly shrewd ear to the reasons each gives for wishing to adopt a child. This may throw a most valuable light upon the vital question about which the adoption society is seeking assurance: is the couple capable of the task which they want to undertake? For husband and wife cannot be a benign influence upon the child unless, mentally and physically, they are sufficiently robust to withstand the pressures which will be involved.

Yet even when assured that a couple would be suitable foster parents, this is not the end of the matter. They are not simply handed the child who is next in the queue. On the contrary, they will have to wait until the adoption society can offer them a child who is likely to make a relationship with these particular foster parents which will be mutually satisfactory.

The arrival of a child will test three fundamental factors in every marriage: the personality of the husband, the personality of the wife, and the link between them. At different times the strain may be on one factor more than another, but the other two can never escape entirely, and if one factor succumbs, then the marriage may be wrecked.

Such an occurrence may undeniably be detrimental to the child, and this aspect of the matter seldom fails to catch the public eye. But it tends to be forgotten that the parents are also people: that they too are in a process of evolution, and that a rupture in their relationship may be a sad and serious obstacle to their progress. This is especially sad if, at the time they proposed to embark upon parenthood, anyone with sufficient insight could have predicted that its demands would be too much for them, and that they should have been encouraged to concentrate further upon all that is implied in strengthening the relationship between themselves.

But in contrast to the rigorous selection procedure to which people who are thoroughly familiar with both sides of the picture deem it necessary to subject prospective foster parents, no steps at all are taken to ensure that the ordinary married couple will be able to withstand the burden which even the most congenial child will inevitably impose upon them. Instead, their fitness for parenthood is taken for granted, and within weeks or months after their marriage they may actually have pressure put upon them to embark upon the operation without delay. A considerable number do so, and the stage for potential disaster is set.

Let us start from the premise that the female body is subject to a recurrent urge to breed. Many a woman never feels better than when she is pregnant, especially with her first child, until the sheer mechanics of advanced pregnancy become obtrusive. Some of her well-being may be due to the fact that during this period her relationship with her husband is probably happier than ever. No matter how much he may have loved his wife before, he will feel especially tender and protective towards her now that she is carrying their child. And the knowledge that ahead of her lies an inescapable event of at least considerable discomfort, and an undeniable element of danger, adds a sense of poignant anxiety.

After the birth, the final phase of the breeding urge is responsible for the many-faceted joy which the mother derives from her infant. And, illogical though it may be, there is a certain pleasure and satisfaction in having achieved fatherhood. For a time the husband cannot do too much for his wife, and neither of them too much for the baby.

Amongst animals in the wild, this final phase persists until the young are capable of fending for themselves. But the human mother is fortunate if it endures to the end of breast-feeding. And it is when these instinctual feelings have subsided in the mother, and the novelty has worn off fatherhood, that for both parents the task of parenthood really begins. This task may be expected to last for a minimum of sixteen years and is never without hazards: for the mother, for the father, and for the link between them.

Now the presence of a baby in the house demands that there is someone on duty for each of the twenty-four hours. But the fact of being the baby's mother does not necessarily equip her with the temperament to fulfill her maternal obligations virtually single-handed, as in these days so many women have to do. For the strains accumulate.

Her sleep will be broken, and an endless series of small crises are liable to interrupt every activity, every attempt at concentrated thought. The demand for regular meals imposes a certain rigidity upon her day. She must resign herself to the fact that unless she has been able to make other arrangements she cannot leave the house without taking the baby with her, and then must set her pace to his.

When the baby becomes mobile she knows she must be ceaselessly watchful to guard against the obvious sources of accidents, open fires, projecting saucepan handles, and so on, but soon she learns that if she takes her eyes off him for a moment he may still contrive to injure himself in some way which had escaped her imagination. A little later she will have to endure endless demands for the favorite story, and stern correction if she misplaces a single word.

Yet such factors touch only the fringe of what is

involved in the care of the most healthy, placid, and congenial baby. I have not touched upon such matters as the feelings of personal inadequacy that may be evoked by periods of crying for which the cause cannot be found and which nothing short of exhaustion seems to abate: feelings which can easily be transformed into anger with the child, and so have to be rigidly suppressed. How easily this transformation can occur I have learned through personal experience.

At about eleven-thirty one night during my first marriage the baby began to cry. Changing her diaper with particular care to see that no pin went astray brought no relief, and the offer of a supplementary bottle was indignantly, not to say contemptuously, brushed aside. Picking her up and carrying her around for half an hour was equally ineffective.

Feeling challenged not only as a father but as a physician, I went to work. I tested the rigidity of her neck for signs of early meningitis. I looked in her mouth for an erupting tooth, and at her throat against the possibility of an infection. I fetched an auriscope and inspected each ear.

Slipping her sleeping suit down to her knees I examined her chest, her abdomen, and to be on the safe side, examined her rectally as well. Satisfied at least that she was neither brewing nor suffering any serious condition I put her back in her cot: but the crying continued until, even more exhausted than I was myself, she fell asleep.

It was during these endless two hours that I realised how easily the inadequacy she was causing me to feel about myself could have been turned into anger against her. I am thankful this did not happen, for in the morning the cause of my ineffectiveness was revealed. I had failed to notice that the elastic on one foot of her sleepingsuit had become wedged between two toes and had caused a deep indentation.

It is no reflection upon a woman's value as a human

being if these frustrations and anxieties, of which she bears the brunt, drive her to the limit of her tolerance. If this limit is exceeded, the result may be a nervous breakdown, which may obviously have disastrous consequences for her and for the family as a whole. But a more insidious danger to her relationship with her husband is that she reaches a state of chronic tiredness in which she is unable to see any pleasure anywhere; of chronic irritation which may cause her to find fault with everyone, especially with her husband.

It will take more sympathy and understanding on his part than many husbands possess if he is not to react defensively and make matters worse. At best he develops around himself a psychological barrier to protect him against his wife's reproaches, and gradually there develops an atmosphere of "his" and "hers"— the antithesis of the "ours" which is the essence of a true marriage.

But there are women, even women who previously had wide intellectual and physical interests, who find that the almost single-handed care of a baby, and the toddler which he soon becomes, is the most rewarding activity of all. For such a woman the danger is that she may become engrossed in her child at the expense of the link with her husband.

He may accept that the baby's paraphernalia are an inevitable addition to the furniture, but it is improbable that he likes it. He may accept that the baby has to be bathed and fed at six o'clock in the evening, and that since his wife cannot be in two places at once he must forego that drink together when he gets home, which used to be one of the happiest features of their day— but he will miss it. He may accept innumerable small ways in which it is the baby who has the first claim on his wife's time and attention. But, and so imperceptibly that he scarcely realises it is happening, he begins to find interests outside the home increasingly attractive.

A drink with an office friend before setting off for home? Well why not—she won't be finished with the baby before seven. The stag party next Saturday to celebrate Joe's promotion? Not a bad idea—I'm sure she won't mind.

And almost certainly she genuinely does not mind, because at this stage she does not recognise the symptom for what it is, and nor, probably, does he. It is all so gradual. There is not the drama of his wife having become infatuated with another man, nor he with another woman. Nor is he consumed with jealousy of the baby. But, perhaps barely consciously, he senses that the essence of the woman whom he married— because to be with her was the dearest thing in life— has withdrawn from him. And so, again scarcely aware of what he is doing, he is adjusting to life without that essence.

Now if both awaken simultaneously to what is happening, the situation can probably be rapidly restored. But too often one, and it does not matter which one, recognises it in advance of the other. And in the frightened, angry reproaches and ripostes which are all too likely to ensue, the relationship between husband and wife may receive a blow from which it never recovers.

To understand the ways in which parents may be vulnerable, it is necessary to consider certain psychological mechanisms which, in varying degrees, are very widespread. Perhaps the most significant is the confusion between being loved and feeling indispensable.

No man who really loved his wife would wish her to be unable to survive adequately if he were to die. Certainly she would be sad, for sadness at parting is the price of happiness in company. But he would abhor the idea that she was dependent on him, for love finds it difficult to flourish except in freedom.

Dependency is a barrier against love. It may make it impossible for the wife to believe her husband stays with her because he really loves her and not merely from a sense of duty. She may hate herself on account of her dependency, but displace these feelings onto her husband, and so, quite irrationally, grow to dislike him. He, for his part, may fear that she only stays with him out of necessity. "You don't *love* me, you only *need* me . . ." is a taunt often flung by a husband or wife in anger. A person who is loved will always be needed: but a person who aims at being indispensable is very unlikely to be loved.

Yet very many people, and often those who use the word "love" most frequently, have lost sight of its real implications, and rely upon the feeling that they are indispensable for an illusion of emotional security. It is a woman who is making this mistake who is liable to revel in the dependency of her child to an extent which endangers the link with her husband. When the child, very properly, becomes absorbed in learning to do things for himself, she may, instead of being delighted with his progress, interpret his increasing independence as a withdrawal of affection. The anxiety which she may then suffer is likely to drive her to become possessive towards her husband, thus causing their relationship to deteriorate still further.

The father is likely to be vulnerable on a different score, through forgetting that his essential contribution was simply the sperm which fertilised the ovum to which the incomer became attached. Obviously the sperm carried certain genes which helped to make it possible for the supra-physical to construct this particular soma, and clearly this soma is an integral factor of the child's personality. But it is easy for the father to fantasise the child as an extension of himself to a degree which is irrational and dangerous.

The source of such fantasies lies outside his awareness, and is usually the unconscious extension of an attempt to make the child compensate for certain respects in which he has felt inferior. These fantasies

171

may interfere with his objective appraisal of the child's potentialities, and cause him to see them through a haze of hopes and fears. When the child reaches a standard, in any respect, which is no higher than any dispassionate observer might have predicted, such a father can suffer a severe blow to his self-esteem. His own feelings of inferiority, of resentment against himself, become inflamed, and, all too probably, will swiftly be transformed into a totally unjustified resentment of the child.

This is particularly liable to happen if the child is slow to learn some skill in which the father takes pride and has been trying to impart. It is entirely justifiable to feel pleased if one has succeeded in teaching someone a skill which will add to their enjoyment of life; and if one has failed to do so it is right to review one's technique as a teacher. But it is entirely unjustifiable to resent the pupil who happens to lack the basic aptitudes which would have enabled him to profit from one's efforts.

A contrary state of affairs sometimes occurs which is unlikely to become apparent until late adolescence. The child when young fulfils all his father's hopes, and his promise nourishes paternal pride. But if the time comes when the child is clearly about to exceed his father's attainments in a particular field, this promise may be seen as a threat, and evoke intense resentment. Such a deplorable situation will never affect the father who has always recognised that the child is an individual with innate potentialities acquired during a long-history.

If either parent harbours unjustified hostility against their child, hostility which expresses itself in unfair treatment or criticism, the other one may try to defend him. But lacking the know-how to resolve the resentment, strife between father and mother deals yet another blow to the relationship between husband and wife. Alternatively the parents may unite against the child in resentment which is unjust, and this shared resentment may become the strongest link between them. But as this link is forged from negative feelings it can never unite them in positive affection.

Parents who recognise that the basic attitudes of their child were acquired by his own efforts, and that he would not have been born, to them or to anyone else, unless at least some of these attitudes needed to be redirected, will not be surprised when they find that certain aspects of his character are unloveable. But if they believe that his unloveability is either inherited through them, or due to their ineptitude as parents, they will inevitably feel guilty, and probably try to foist their guilt on each other. The needless guilt feelings of many parents would be substantially relieved if they could see their child with true insight.

I have had many patients who initially presented a convincing picture of having been the victim of parents who were over-protective and dominating, or who rejected them, or who failed to teach them self-discipline. But as their stories unfolded it became clear that the child with the dominating parents had been only too glad to be relieved of the necessity to think for himself; that the rejected child had merely been unsuccessful in claiming his mother's undivided attention; and that the discontented rebel had been a bully from the start.

The time will probably come when the child leaves home to start life on his own. Ideally, the regret which the parents feel at his absence will be tempered by the fact that they are now free fully to enjoy the link between each other, which has been growing steadily stronger through the years. But for parents who allowed the child to be an obstruction to the development of their link, this may be a critical event.

If the child has been the cause of frank hostility between them, he also served as something of a buffer. Now the buffer has gone: but the hostility remains. A

173

somewhat similar result may ensue from a different cause: if the child provided a convenient target upon which the parents could project hostility that arose within themselves about each other, they will have been able to evade the real source of their hostility. But in so doing they deprived themselves of the chance of resolving it, and with the disappearance of the target are left with no one to snipe at but each other.

If their interest in the child has constituted their principal link, they may find when he goes that they are facing each other almost as strangers. Unless they have the courage to admit the situation, and an urgent desire, even at this late stage, to start to create a true love relationship, they may very easily drift into separate lives which have little genuine overlap.

The difficulties which can arise from this are not going to be made easier as automation extends, giving people greater leisure and forcing down the age of retirement. It will presumably be several years before society has adjusted to the problems which this will create.

The feeling of usefulness which a man derives from his job should be only one of the factors that contribute to his self-esteem: of at least equal importance to him should be the regard in which he can justifiably feel he is held by his wife. Lacking this, when his job comes to an end he must either quickly find some new way in which he can feel he is pulling his weight; or face a serious crisis.

His wife will probably have contrived a way of life which at least gives her the illusion of being fully occupied; but he is unlikely to wish to share in her chosen activities, even if she wanted him to do so. Under these circumstances it is not surprising if he develops a severe depression, and one which is difficult to treat. It may not be at all easy for him to find a satisfactory occupation; and one can neither truthfully reassure him that he is of vital importance to his wife, nor give him back the years which he might have lived more wisely.

If he avoids going into a depression, he may, especially if funds permit, find some hobby, some form of activity, which enjoyably occupies his time. But if he fails to do so, boredom or loneliness may cause him to form a sincere attachment to another woman. This would not matter, any more than it would matter if his wife became attached to another man, if these two events occurred simultaneously; but they rarely do so. Thus the one who is threatened with being left, faced with the prospect of loss of prestige, refuses to accept an end to the farce of their marriage, and instead of wishing the other a benign "God speed," begins a war of attrition which may persist until they are divorced by death.

In the course of this attrition both parties tend to become embittered with life in general. Their capacities for bearing grudges, for seeking revenge, for feeling jealousy, and indulging the other corrosive attitudes increase through constant exercise; and so they reach the grave as two thoroughly soured personalities.

Now if their death were followed by the extinction of the personality, such lives would have been sad enough; but in fact, to the best of my understanding, the implications are far more serious. Instead of resolving the relevant problems in their personalities they have added to them; for one must always remember that the sour oldster is only too likely to reappear as a sour baby.

It may be objected that I have painted too gloomy a picture of the hazards of parenthood; that it must be biased because, as a psychiatrist, the majority of people I see are those who have succumbed to stress, and that the couples whose lives have been infinitely enriched by their children have passed me by.

It is true that in this chapter I have not been concerned with the joys of parenthood, for these have been publicised often enough. It is also true that I have never been asked for an appointment by a stranger who was enjoying life to the full and felt a sudden urge to drop in and tell me so. A psychiatrist, however, does not spend his entire life in his consulting room; in the course of each year he probably makes as many social contacts as anyone else. But while he can switch off any tendency to look at people with a professional eye, he cannot avoid being aware of certain nuances of speech and behaviour which might escape someone with a different training.

Assuming that my account of the hazards of parenthood is not exaggerated, what practical suggestions arise?

In the first place, prospective parents should strive to contemplate the undertaking purely intellectually. They must appreciate that as our society becomes ever more complex, the trials of parenthood become more difficult and more prolonged.

Technology is advancing so rapidly that the time which a young man or woman may be compelled to spend in the capacity of a student is constantly increasing, while subjects of which the father knew nothing may be part of the curriculum of a schoolboy. This is one of the factors which tend to cause the young, rightly or wrongly, to hold their parents in scant respect, and to be insusceptible to the dubious weapon of parental authority.

If the parents are wise ones, the children, in due course, may echo the sentiments of Mark Twain, who said in effect that when he left home at seventeen he thought his father was an old fool, but when he came back at twenty-three he was astonished to find how much the old man had learned in the meantime.

But it may not be easy for a couple to take a dispassionate view of their potentialities as parents in face of the various influences which may be brought to bear on them. If they show no signs of producing a child after two or three years of marriage, they may evoke either suspicion that all is not well between them, or mutterings that they are failing in their "Duty to Society." In view of the universal alarm over the population explosion it is difficult to imagine what this duty is supposed to be. But that this totally unrealistic feeling persists is shown by the fact that couples who have demonstrated their ability to breed are accorded a status which tends to be denied to the childless. In fact a child is often seen as a status symbol of the parents' adulthood and of their worth as citizens. I have even known couples who frankly admitted that they had a child only so as not to feel outdone by their neighbours.

Potential grandparents are another source of pressure which urges a young couple to start a family without delay. On two occasions, during the wedding reception I have heard the bride's mother express the hope that there would be "a baby on the way" before the end of the honeymoon. In one instance I have little doubt that this ill-considered hope represented the mother's reaction to the void that would be caused by her daughter's departure; in the other I think it was based on a muddleheaded belief that a child would necessarily cement the marriage.

The pressure exerted by potential grandparents on a son is usually not so immediate, but sooner or later they may demand from him an heir to "carry on the line." An heir may have financial advantages, in cases of entailed property, but is otherwise of very little significance since the most that can be perpetuated is a certain number of physical characteristics—a far too trivial reason for encouraging a couple to embark on a task for which they may be quite unsuited.

A variation for the longing for heirs is a hazy notion that descendants are a kind of passport to immortality. This, of course, is nonsense: immortality lies within oneself. Obviously we all hope to be remembered with affection by the people we know, but the fact of blood relationship makes this neither more likely nor more valuable.

I cannot emphasise too strongly that the arrival of a child does not necessarily strengthen the benign link between a couple. On the contrary, it may distort this link beyond repair or even turn it into fetters. It takes both time and effort to develop a link which is sufficiently strong to be burnished, instead of corroded, by parenthood; so it would be a step in the right direction if it became a social gaffe to start a baby during the first two years of marriage.

There is no reason whatever why a couple should feel obliged to have a child. There are already too many people in the world, and if there is a genius waiting to come in, there will never be a shortage of fertilised ova from which he can choose. In developing their relationship with one another a couple may well be doing all that in this particular lifetime they have set out to do; and a couple who radiate their happiness are an asset to the community of incalculable value.

So far I have tried to outline the motives for having a child which, from the standpoint of the prospective parents, I view with concern. One could summarise these motives by saying that any couple are in danger if they are relying upon gaining from their child whatsoever.

I know very well that they may gain a great deal. They may gain his sincere appreciation of what they have done for him, and his permanent affection. They may gain profound gratification from having contributed to the development of an individual who makes very many people thankful that he was born. But the hard fact is that even the most wise and loving parents may get nothing except the satisfaction of knowing that they performed a task to the best of their ability.

I am sure that it is important for parents to realise

that their child does not owe them anything; it is not incumbent upon him to make any return for what he has received from them. His duty lies in handing on what they taught him to other children—including his own if he sees fit to have any, and to the world at large.

Lest I seem to be emphasising that parenthood entails great sacrifices, let me explain that this is in no way my intention. A doctor may grumble, "I was called out of bed three times last week and the week before that I had to miss the last act of an enthralling play." But even before he embarked on his career he knew that such things would inevitably happen. If he finds that he is beginning to think in terms of sleep "sacrificed," or a theatre "sacrificed," then he is no longer where his heart is and would be well advised to seek a different niche.

Parenthood, no less than medicine, will impose a pattern of life upon its practitioners; and if a couple foresee aspects of this pattern as involving "sacrifices," they would be wiser not to embark upon it.

Modern parents have abjectly accepted more blame for the shortcomings of their offspring than was their due. This was an inevitable consequence of allegiance to a philosophy which failed to recognise that every individual is responsible for the quality of his own character. Failing this recognition, it was natural enough for psychiatry to assume that a personality is predominantly an expression of the influences brought to bear upon it by the grownups, and, most notably, the parents. In truth, the parents can do no more than help a child to modify the character which he brought with him: to reinforce his benign aspects, and to change those attitudes which are diverting his energies from the course of his evolution. This is the essence of parenthood—bringing a child up; as opposed to breeding, which is merely bringing one down.

In the absence of a Board of Examiners to ensure that

a couple is qualified for the task, there are some questions which all prospective parents should ask themselves. For instance, "Have we ourselves grown up? Have we resolved all childish attachments to our own parents?"

A couple who are still emotionally dependent on their parents are liable either to try to make their child conform to the standards of behaviour which were imposed upon themselves, or else to fall over backwards to protect him from similar pressures. Whichever course they pursue, their treatment of him is likely to be inconsistent and often inappropriate. Only when they can see their parents through adult eyes will they be able to recognise which aspects of their own childhood they wish to hand on, and which should be scrupulously avoided.

I have learned in the consulting room that if a patient who is adult in years spontaneously uses some variant of "Mummy" or "Daddy," as opposed to the socially or biologically descriptive "my mother" or "my father," there is nearly always a residual dependency which is a source of trouble.

Such a patient, a man in his thirties, was a father speaking about the undue irritation he felt for his six-year-old son. He was complaining that the boy was too babyish, and by way of illustration was describing how, on the previous day, the boy, after falling down, had run bawling to his "mummy." But in telling the story, he also made a slip of the tongue. Instead of saying "the boy ran to *his* mummy," he said, "the boy ran to my mummy," and this was the key to the whole situation. A considerable portion of the personality of this man—in many ways a most competent citizen was seeing his wife as a mother-figure, and resenting the son as though he were a rival baby, playing expertly upon the mother's sympathies. Only when this man had resolved this infantile aspect of himself did he become capable of being an effective parent.

Not long ago, a merry girl of nineteen was enthusing about her forthcoming marriage, and prattling happily of her intention to start a baby without delay. Her prospective husband had raised no objection, and she added, "Daddy will be simply thrilled."

I next learned that on her bed she kept the doll which she had had since the nursery, and her attachment to this object was a further indication of her reluctance to relinquish her childhood. Finally, when I asked her position in the family hierarchy, she replied with another phrase which experience has taught me is ominous, "I am the baby!" I was relieved to hear, a few weeks later, that her engagement had ended. Because what she really wanted was a living doll to drool over.

An infant who becomes incorporated into the mother's narcissistic fantasies is liable to develop the "Never-had-it-so-good" syndrome. The essence of this is that the child is led so to overvalue babyhood that he never wants to relinquish it. Having been deluged with adulation merely because he happens to be a baby, he is likely to resist being prompted to enter the next phase, in which he has to play a more active role in order to justify his existence.

Another aspect of the same syndrome is that someone who, during early childhood, has become accustomed to an unduly lavish measure of praise and attention may become very anxious when, in new surroundings, he is accorded no more than he merits. This may lead him constantly to seek notice and approval in a way which earns him dislike. Therefore he is very likely, and with good reason, to lack self-confidence. He may try to hide his insecurity beneath a façade of brash assurance, or else develop feelings of inadequacy to a degree which is crippling.

The next question is whether the prospective mother has any irrational fears about pregnancy or childbirth, for she should take steps to have any such fears allayed rather than embark upon maternity in a spirit of gallantry. I say "irrational" fears, because these are far more likely to be picked up by the fœtus than fears based on public opinion or economics, and can be tantamount to a voice perpetually shouting at him, "I do not want you—your presence terrifies me."

I think it highly probable, although this has yet to be proved, that the prevailing mood of the mother is reflected in the details of the micro-chemistry of her blood. So if she spends her pregnancy in a state of chronic fear, subtle changes in her blood may induce feelings of disease in the unborn child. Experience suggests that if he feels that his presence is genuinely welcome, he can take such hazards as motor accidents and air raids without suffering the slightest physical or psychological damage. Many patients, regressed to the later weeks of intrauterine life, have relived sensations which were caused by sexual intercourse between the parents. If this is performed gently, and affords the mother pleasure, I believe it is thoroughly beneficial for the fœtus. On the other hand, if the mother is submitting to the act only under duress, he is very liable to interpret the event as an assault upon himself, which may well increase any fears he already has that the world which awaits him is a hostile place.

If a mother becomes pregnant merely to gratify needs of her own—to boost her ego or to render her position with her husband more secure, it is as though her feelings, being concerned primarily with herself, bypass the incomer, who is left out in the emotional cold. As a result, he feels intensely lonely, and after he is born, this may be a factor in causing him to develop very slowly. Aware of his mother's essential lack of interest, he fears that instead of giving him time to acquire self-reliance, she may withdraw her support when he shows only the first signs of independence. Therefore he fears to go forward, and seeks to bind her to him with his helplessness.

When I became convinced of the reality of reincarnation, I realised that the importance I had attached to prenatal experiences had been exaggerated. But the fact remains that it is a period of no less psychological significance than any other, and therefore the last thing a responsible parent wishes to do is to provide a prenatal environment in which the child is likely to feel unwanted or endangered. The effect of this could only be to reinforce the unhealthy traits in his character which were at least part of the motive for his incarnation.

The event of birth, even a birth which the obstetrician would cheerfully describe as "uncomplicated" and the mother as "easy," is a frightening ordeal for the infant. Presumably the most accomplished trapeze-artist is not entirely free of apprehension each time he risks his life; and similarly the infant, although he has experienced innumerable successful births, is still aware that each one is a hazard. Experience with patients suggests that the infant knows he must be born just as clearly as we know that we have to die, and he may or may not feel ready for the adventure. I recall one woman, regressed to the period immediately prior to birth, who exclaimed indignantly, "But it is Me who should say when I want to be born!" She had been a brow presentation, and appeared to recall deliberately moving her head into this position in an effort to resist the process; which it did, very effectively, because instead of her head presenting its smallest diameter to squeeze through the birth-canal, it presented almost its greatest.

It would seem that if the intra-uterine period has been ideal, from the point of view of the fœtus, he feels confident of surviving birth, and is actually looking forward to the wider, independent life which lies ahead. But if, rightly or wrongly, he has felt himself to be under attack throughout this time, then he sees the expulsive forces of birth, which are entirely outside his control, as an attempt to thrust him into extinction.

So many patients have stressed the pain caused by the impact of noise and light immediately after being born that I am sure it is desirable to reduce these as far as possible. Voices should be hushed and the clatter of instruments on stone floors, the banging of doors and so forth, should be avoided.

It would be a kindly gesture to reduce the lighting as the baby's head is on the point of emerging; and in order to mitigate the feeling of loneliness and separation, which seems to be one of the most painful of all the aspects of birth, the baby should be placed naked against the naked chest of the mother. A screen arranged across the waist of the mother would then shield the baby when the lights are restored to full power so that the technical aspects of the delivery can be completed.

The baby can be given its first bath at leisure, but then should be returned to naked contact with the mother. Skin to skin contact is such a vital means of transmitting a feeling of security to a baby that far more use should be made of it, especially during feeding. I believe it is also important that the baby should always be within sound of a friendly adult. The custom which prevails in some maternity establishments of allowing the babies to howl their heads off unattended in a separate nursery has nothing to recommend it.

Several patients have relived, with acute distress, being held upside-down by the ankles and slapped. Any manœuvres necessary to help the baby to breathe should be performed with the utmost gentleness: the weight of forceps dangling from the newly severed umbilical cord can make a baby feel he is being eviscerated.

There can be no greater mistake than to believe that an infant is ever "too young to notice." As I have tried to point out, he is able to notice and to register everything: but as he lacks sufficient intellectual equipment to interpret the event, or to understand the reason for it, he is liable to react to anything which causes him pain as though it were a deliberate assault.

This was well illustrated by a patient, a man in his forties, who returned to consciousness after his first session under hypnosis, rubbing his lower lip and complaining that it was tingling. The sensation soon subsided, but recurred on nearly every occasion that hypnosis was used.

The patient had told me, when I was taking his case history, that at birth he had been unable to suck and so, when he was two weeks old, his adenoids had been removed. Later in his treatment he suddenly regressed spontaneously to early infancy. With his mouth wide open as though fixed by a gag, his head rolled wildly as he emitted inarticulate grunts of distress. He was able to splutter, "They are hurting my throat!" But when I asked, "Why are they doing that?" he blurted, "To stop me taking my bottle!"

As he uttered these words he wrenched himself out of hypnosis and exclaimed, "My God! How on earth could I have said that!" Then, rubbing his lip with the familiar gesture he added, "That explains the tingling in my lip. It was something to do with the operation.

I am convinced that infantile circumcision can be a potent psychological trauma. Assuming that the individual begins each incarnation without an unconscious, this operation is a powerful stimulus to construct one without delay.

In the first place, even if perception of pain is not at its peak during infancy, the infliction of this mutilation is an agonising barbarity. Very naturally the child holds his parents responsible for the assault, but because he realises that they are also the people upon whom his survival depends, this invokes more anxiety than he can tolerate. So he thrusts his fear of his parents into his unconscious, whence it may reappear as a deep mistrust of the world in general, a resolve never to be cheated again, and a determination to "get his own back."

In addition, even the most balanced personality is likely to have had an incarnation in which sex was associated with grief, or guilt, or fear, and nothing can be more calculated to arouse these latent memories, and attach them to his current sexual development, than such an attack upon his sexual organ.

Anyone who had seen patients reliving their circumcision would share my conviction that it should never be performed except when there is a clear surgical indication that it is unavoidable.

Another question which prospective parents should consider is whether they would be sufficiently clear-sighted to discern the real motives underlying various facets of their child's behaviour. Obviously I do not share the view that the personality of a child is an unorganised collection of anti-social impulses awaiting civilisation, but it would be unrealistic to suggest that he will not have a number of basic attitudes which he needs to change. If the parents fail to recognise these attitudes—and they may be concealed beneath the most beguiling behaviour, then they are simply allowing the child to reinforce those aspects of his character for which he will increasingly dislike himself.

But to recognise a child's unacceptable aspects is only the first step. The next is to inspire him with the wish to change them. Fear may change what a person does; but not what he wants to do. The only effective agent the parents can use to bring about their child's voluntary redirection of his energies is the filial affection and respect they have earned from him. To earn these they will require a capacity for wise leadership.

What is leadership? Surely, it is a quality developed by a personality who, for a very long time, has been determined to exercise his power of choice, and has had the moral courage to act upon his decisions. When a potential leader is seen to be moving with the crowd it is because, on this occasion, his choice coincides with that of the majority, and not because it is the popular decision. Similarly, when he is moving contrary to the crowd, it is because his choice differs from theirs, and not because he wishes to stand out from the crowd or to rebel against it.

As a result of always making his own decisions, and the experience he has gained through acting upon them, he is able to make up his mind more quickly and more wisely than people who have had less practice. Thus, more and more frequently, he is the person who moves first. When the day comes that other people choose to follow him, he has become a leader.

Every time that parents are hoodwinked by a child, or caused to reverse a decision as a result of his nuisance value, they become smaller in his eyes, and their capacity to help him is reduced. Obviously even the most admirable parents will not always be right, but if they frankly admit their error this evidence of human fallibility in no way diminishes the child's respect.

Far from agreeing with the widely held view that a child must never be made to feel rejected, I believe that under certain circumstances rejection is a very right and very effective policy. Nothing is more likely to cause him to wish to change an aspect of himself than the realisation that someone whom he loves and admires finds it absolutely unacceptable. A couple who have learned to love each other possess the best qualifications for teaching a child that love has to be earned, by being loveable.

9

AN ASSORTMENT OF APPARITIONS
by Joan Grant

I have never seen a traditional ghost, the amorphous, faintly luminous figure, which glides through the precincts and then suddenly vanishes. My failure to do so has sometimes offended the owners of haunted houses, who have reacted to my inability to see their family phantom as they might have done had I refused to inspect their new baby.

The apparitions I have encountered seemed so substantial that it was sometimes difficult to recognise that they were not solid. When I was a child, mistakes of this nature frequently got me into trouble, so I usually pretended not to see strangers until I had made sure that they were visible to everyone else. I am still apt to forget that second-sight is an extension of normal vision, just as I sometimes forget that Denys, because he is red-green color blind, cannot share my enthusiasm for the scarlet blaze of a field of poppies.

The first time I remember causing a family row by failing to realise that a visitor belonged in the category of They-who-should-not-be-mentioned occurred when I was five. My father was then a fanatical atheist, and was liable to lock himself in his study if a cleric managed to infiltrate his defences. Even a Church of England clergyman had a high rarity rating, so meeting a Roman Catholic priest, who had come to visit an ailing guest, was a memorable event. His cassock and four-cornered hat with a bobble on top seemed odd enough, but he had the added glory of a facial frill of red whiskers at which I gazed entranced, while, in a rich Irish brogue, he told me that his name was Canon Daly and that his church was in Havant, five miles from my home, Seacourt on Hayling Island.

I did not see him again until two years later, when he came into my bedroom while I was waiting for my parents to come to say good night. I recognised him immediately, because his whiskers were gleaming in the light which streamed through the open doorway. He stood smiling down at me, and I knew he was pleased that I remembered him. I was trying to decide whether to address him as Canon Daly, or as "Father," which an Irish housemaid had told me was the correct title for a priest, when he nodded, as though assuring himself that a job had been done, and walked briskly out of the room without saying anything.

I had either forgotten the anti-cleric taboo or pre-sumed it had been lifted, so I mentioned his visit at breakfast next morning. Father flung down his napkin and strode up to Mother's bedroom. He forgot to shut the door, so I heard him saying, "If you insist on the place being invaded by ecclesiastics you will kindly inform me, so that I can keep out of their way. But I'm damned if I will have them creeping about the house like black beetles! The R.C. incumbent from Havant actually had the impertinence to go up to Joan's room last night!"

I had already had too much experience of being used as ammunition, by either or both contestants, during a parental argument; so I withdrew to a hideout in the shrubbery.

There was no further mention of Canon Daly until the following week. Then Mother told me that she had telephoned to his church and found out that he had returned to Ireland eighteen months earlier. So she had written to his new address and had now received the news that he had died on the evening he had come to see me.

"I wonder why he bothered to come here . . . we hardly knew him," I said. "I should have thought he would have had far more exciting things to do now that he's dead."

"He came to see me, not you," said Mother. "I remember telling him that death would prove to him that most of his dogmatic ideas were nonsense, and he promised to come to tell me if he discovered that I was right."

Another occasion when I failed to notice that a visitor had no physical body occurred in 1916. By that stage of the war there were usually about half a dozen wounded officers convalescing at Seacourt. I was particularly fond of one of them, a major in the Rifle Brigade, who had to lie face-downwards in his spinal carriage, which I helped to push round the garden, because most of his buttocks had been blown off. Shell splinters were still working their way out of the wound, and he gave me one of them as a souvenir. He was getting much better when suddenly he had a serious relapse through developing acute sepsis. I had not been allowed to see him for several days, and then I heard that he was to have an emergency operation. This would be done in one of the bedrooms, hung with sheets dipped in disinfectant, as in those days operations often took place at home instead of the patient being moved to a hospital.

I happened to be in the hall when the doctors arrived. I knew two of them, the surgeon and his partner, who was to give the anæsthetic, but the third man was a stranger. I presumed he was another doctor, so was mildly surprised that instead of wearing formal black clothes like the other two he had on a blue coat with gold buttons. As I watched him walking upstairs the buttons glinted in the sunlight and I noticed the crest on them.

I must have mentioned him to Mother, because the next time I was allowed to visit the major he asked me to describe the man who had come with the two doctors who had operated on him. When I mentioned the blue coat with the crested buttons the major said, "I am glad he still wears his favourite coat. It was blue like his hunt uniform, and had his crest, as you noticed, on a set of gold buttons . . . very observant of you to notice that they were not brass. He was the M.F.H. of his own pack of hounds, when we still had our family place in Yorkshire."

He paused and stared out of the window. Then he said, "He has come to give me a hand on two other occasions when I was in a tricky situation. The first time was when I had black-water fever in the Belgian Congo, and the second was when I nearly chucked in my hand after getting this packet in my backside."

He smiled. "If you look in my stud-box—it's in the top drawer of the dressing table, you will find one of my father's buttons. I cut it off the blue coat he was buried in, just before they closed his coffin . . . fifteen years ago."

Seeing such ghosts as the canon and the major's father was in no way disquieting; in fact they were far more welcome visitors than the chattering flocks in the drawing-room, who were only too likely to demand a goodnight kiss instead of being placated with a curtsey. But I was now becoming closely concerned with people who had so recently been killed that they had not yet realised they were safely dead. I knew that as soon as I was asleep, instead of being a child I would again be a responsible adult, who had been allotted a specific kind of "war work." This work consisted of convincing men who had died in battle that they had no reason to fear dying, for this familiar transition which they had so needlessly dreaded had already taken place.

Sometimes this proved to be easy, and I woke happy in the knowledge of a job well done. But if I had been sent to help someone who had allowed dogma to infect him with grotesque terrors, or who had clung to the agonies which had affected his physical body because he thought them the only alternative to oblivion, the task of releasing him could be arduous. These experiences were as vivid as if they had occurred on the three-dimensional level of reality, so it was difficult to endure their impact on the component of my personality which was still confined by the intellectual equipment of a young child. Sometimes the memory of sensations would persist for several minutes after I knew I was awake, and the stench of gangrene often caused me to vomit. I went through a period when I was so afraid of the terrors associated with sleep that to postpone it I would sit on the cold parquet which surrounded my nursery carpet, or tweak out hairs, or hold my eyelids open, or drive an orange stick deeply under my nails.

As everyone who has encountered similar realities knows only too well, this type of work entails so intimate a degree of identification with the other person that instead of feeling, "This is happening to him," one feels, "This is happening to me." So I would wake feeling that it was I who had been entangled in barbed-wire, or had been trying to cram glistening coils back into my belly, or drowning in mud, or choking with phosgene gas.

These hazards, which I now know to be an occupational risk which must be accepted by anyone who chooses this particular profession, would have been more tolerable had I been able to talk about them. I tried to do so, but when told not to invent such horrible stories I presumed that my description had not been sufficiently vivid to carry conviction and so added further macabre details. This caused my parents to decide that for some unknown reason I had started to suffer from nightmares. For my mother expected the dead to approach the living circumspectly, preferably through the automatic writing of a professional medium; and my father was at that time convinced that the dead stayed dead, and that any alternative theory was mumbo-jumbo.

Their attempts to solve my problems were, from my point of view, exceedingly inept. Any mention of the war was forbidden if I was present, newspapers were whisked out of sight when I entered the room, and a united conspiracy was put into operation which was intended to convince me that the many friends who had already been killed had all died painlessly with a bullet through the forehead.

This conspiracy was so effective that I began to wonder if they had a firmer grasp of reality than I had: in which case I was undoubtedly mad. However, these speculations about my own sanity—and even at that age I had recognised that sanity is the ability to see things as they really are, lasted only for a few days, and were relieved by a collection of photographs, which amply confirmed that the conditions I knew through true-dreaming were in no way imaginary.

These photographs had been brought to the house by Glory Hancock, a cousin-by-marriage from North Carolina, who had taken them while working as a theatre-sister in casualty clearing stations. She was on her way to the United States, where she intended to use them to raise money for the Red Cross. Her son Westray, who was two years older than I, told me about them, adding in a whisper that they were so horrific that his mother kept them locked in one of her suitcases because they upset even the most robust grown-ups. As he knew where to find the keys it was easy to borrow the photographs while our parents were at dinner. Certainly they were terrible, for the wounds were only covered, if covered at all, with field dressings, and the patients in no way resembled those photographed neatly arrayed in hospital beds. There were men without eyes, without noses, without more than a vestige of their original faces. There were also corpses stacked like cord wood along the wall of a barn: and a much worse photograph of the same scene, on the back of which Glory had written, "Three days later. After the rats."

Had I had the cooperation of a sympathetic adult I might have collected some interesting evidence of extrasensory perception during this period, but only one incident survives, and that through the confidence I suddenly felt in one of the convalescent officers with whom I happened to be alone at breakfast. I told him that during the night I had been helping a man called McAndrew, who had been so painlessly killed that he thought he had only been struck by a spent bullet which could not have even bruised his chest. I did not know the name of his regiment, but described the badge on his uniform. I also gave the slang name for the sector of the frontline trench in which he had waited before going on his last patrol into no-man's-land.

My confidant took considerable trouble to check this information. He then wrote to my father, relating what I had told him and pointing out that it would be difficult to explain away the fact that our conversation had occurred three hours after a battalion of a Canadian regiment, whose badge I had accurately described, had mounted a dawn patrol, from a sector whose slang name I had given, and that the only fatal casualty had been a private soldier called McAndrew.

I was not told about this letter until several years later, for my parents considered it would have encouraged me to talk about my "nightmares," by which time this type of true-dream seldom occurred, probably because with the cessation of mass slaughter it was no

194

longer necessary to use volunteers who still had immature physical bodies.

The first time I engaged in a similar activity when fully awake was in my early twenties, while Leslie and I, together with another young couple, were driving to Austria for a summer holiday. As we wanted to see the castles of the Rhine on our outward journey we went via Brussels, and arrived at the Palace Hotel in time for a late dinner. The hotel was crowded, so we had no choice of accommodation and were allotted rooms on the fifth floor overlooking the service courtyard. I took an illogical dislike to our room, and on the pretext that it was airless, vulnerable to the smell of dustbins outside the kitchens, and had hideous wallpaper, I tried to make Leslie find us another one. Very reasonably he refused, on the grounds that we were only staying overnight and that instead of complaining I ought to be thankful that we had a private bathroom.

After dinner the other three went off to a nightclub, but I was tired and decided to go to bed. While opening the French windows I looked down at the pool of light streaming from the service doors on the ground floor, which seemed so far below me that it was like looking at the reflection in the bottom of a deep well. Outside the windows, which opened inwards, there was a ledge too narrow to be termed a balcony, fenced with ornamental ironwork. Suddenly I clutched the rail, dizzy with vertigo.

I had a long, hot bath. But instead of feeling relaxed I was becoming increasingly tense. In bed I tried to read, but after about half an hour, finding I was unable to concentrate, I switched off the light. I was still very wide awake when suddenly a young man rushed out of the bathroom, and before I had time either to move or speak he flung himself out of the window.

I dived under the bedclothes, so that I should not hear the dreadful thud of his body hitting the paving-stones. After a couple of minutes I forced myself to sit up and listen. But I heard nothing: no agonised groans... no shrieks from the kitchen. So no one could have seen him fall. At least I must shout for someone to help him.

Clutching the handrail I peered down . . . but there was no corpse there. And where the corpse should have been, a waiter was carrying a crate of bottles. This was the first time I had found myself alone in a room which was being haunted by a suicide. If I prayed hard enough someone would come to look after him and then I should stop being so terrified. I prayed until the sweat ran down my forehead: and then got back into bed and tried to sleep.

But I still had my eyes open when the same dreadful sequence was repeated. This time I made myself listen, but I heard nothing; so I was unable to learn whether he had lingered screaming or died instantly.

The obvious thing to do would have been to get dressed, and go for a walk, or try to find the others, or sit in a bar, but this did not occur to me. Praying hadn't helped the poor man, so freeing him from the despair in which he was trapped was a job that I was expected to do. My heart was pounding so hard that it was difficult to think clearly. I had freed many newly dead people while I was asleep . . . but I had been able to do so because I had managed not to be affected by their fear. I could feel his panic soaking into me like ink into blotting-paper. I should have to feel what he was feeling before I could get close enough to him to be of any real help . . . but then his fear might be stronger than my dwindling courage . . . my body might follow his on that horrifying plunge.

At least I could guard against this danger by pulling the chest-of-drawers across the window, so that what-ever happened I could not fall out. When this barrier was in place I felt a little braver, but could only just hold back the waves of fear which I knew would get much more insistent when I attained the necessary degree of identification.

Unless someone is with me, to whom I can describe my feelings while they are occurring, I can seldom remember more than a blurred outline of what I experience during this very difficult type of level-shift. But I know that I shared that man's fall. As he leaned over the balustrade he suddenly tried to regain his balance . . . but it was too late. He tried to thrust out his arms to break his fall . . . he seemed to fall so slowly . . . so slowly. . . . Then he realised that he would be terribly injured, and tried to pull back his arms so as to land on his head. He felt no pain . . . only a grinding thud . . . and then he was back in the bathroom and running towards the window again . . . over and over again . . . over and over again.

I found myself standing with my hands stretched upwards, saying aloud, "Your fear has entered into me and you are free . . . your fear has entered into me and you are free."

The fear, both his and mine, began to release itself in a flood of tears, and sobbing so violent that it bordered on hysteria. Within half an hour I would have been perfectly normal again. Unfortunately for Leslie, he came back when I was in the full spate of the abreaction. He was accused of being a monster who had deliberately left his wife to deal with a suicide . . . it was no thanks to him that I had not broken my neck. . . . The other couple, acutely embarrassed, scuttled off to their room further along the corridor.

Leslie tried to pacify me by saying that I had only had a nightmare. He apologised for this next morning, after discovering from the manager that the previous occupant of our room had thrown himself from the window five days earlier.

It was in June 1956, and I was married to Charles, when I encountered a suicide at the Abbey of Fontevrault, near Saumur in the valley of the Loire.

Fontevrault would have remained for me no more

than a pleasant setting in which to walk off lunch, if we had not come to a high, forbidding wall where a notice beside a pair of enormous iron gates curtly ordered: "SONNEZ LE GUIDE!" On a sudden hunch I obeyed, to regret it a moment later when one of the doors opened to reveal a sinister man in the uniform of a prison warder.

I attempted to retreat, which made him look even more surly. And I was still wondering how to convince him that I was not trying to smuggle a hacksaw to an incarcerated chum by the time he was locking and barring the doors behind us. We were now in a tunnel which, so thick were the outer walls, could easily have garaged a double-decker bus.

"You will wait here until another warder comes to show you round," announced our gaoler. "Visitors are not allowed to circulate except under strict surveillance."

The last thing I wanted to do was to see round a prison, and I said so. His eyes became even more glacial. "You must have wanted to see round the abbey. Otherwise, why did you ring the bell?"

Before I could reply, he withdrew to his lair in the side of the tunnel, slammed the door, and stood staring malevolently through the barred window. A notice informed us that we were in the precincts of an abbey founded at the end of the eleventh century, in which for seven hundred years, until Napoleon turned it into a civil prison, a community of both monks and nuns was ruled over by an abbess. Ahead of us there was an open space of gravel flanked by high curved walls, and at the far side of it a steel door was set in an even higher wall. The only sign of life was three rosebushes, but they were not cheerful either, being smothered with greenfly. So we sat disconsolately on a plank bench in the shade of the tunnel, until after about a quarter of an hour Charles rapped on the door of the gaoler's lair and asked how much longer we were expected to wait.

The door opened a couple of inches to vent: "Twenty minutes—perhaps longer—do not be impatient!"—and then slammed shut again before we could use the delay as an excuse to escape.

I was far more uneasy than circumstances justified. I told myself that I was restless only because I was bored. But my feeling intensified, until I had to admit that there was a ghost in the immediate vicinity. A ghost in a French prison seemed only too probable, and it was the last thing I wanted to see. In an attempt to tune it out I did sums in my head, and then tried to remember the numbers of all the roads we had been on since Le Havre: but these evasions were ineffective.

Reluctantly I had to accept the fact that something, or someone, who five minutes ago had been outside my range of perception, was relentlessly coming into focus. . . . Now I could see three dead men lying on the gravel, near the right-hand wall. There was another man on the ground near them; but he was not dead, for he was trying to crawl. I could smell blood, and cordite—and fear. The stench of fear was sickeningly strong.

With an effort I jerked myself back and said urgently: "Get me out of here or I'll throw up!"

Charles was usually more than willing to help me dodge ghosts, but he said that he felt there was a job here which urgently needed doing. He already had a notebook open on the bench beside him, so I knew I must have been talking aloud instead of only seeing in silence. Trivial fears, of making a scene in public, of being arrested as a dangerous lunatic by the warder, of returning to find myself being stared at by a crowd of giggling tourists, dwindled as I accepted someone else's much deeper fear which I must try to do something about.

I shut my eyes, and started to see what had happened immediately before the men had been killed. But the scene was still impersonal, as though I were watching a coloured film. I could hear myself talking, but it sounded unreal, as though it were being played back on a tape recorder. . . .

"I can see four prisoners—French prisoners. One of them is quite young; the others are middle-aged; but none of them is the ghost. With them is a German guard, a boy of nineteen, with yellow hair and pale blue eyes. He is afraid of the prisoners, although he is armed with a machine-pistol and they have only wooden rakes. They are raking up straw and shavings which fell from the lorries, the lorries which unload here. . . .

"The Frenchmen are whispering to each other; loud whispers which they intend the German boy to over-hear. They describe what will happen to Germans when the town is liberated. The boy tries to ignore them. He wants to shout at them to be silent; but he knows that to do so would betray his fear. He is becoming hysterical with fear. A muscle is twitching in his left eyebrow. But none of the Frenchmen realise they are driving him too far for their own safety. . . .

"Suddenly he shrieks at them to be silent. They grin and go on raking the gravel. The gritty noise of their raking is the only sound. Then they start whispering again. The boy's voice is shrill with fear as he shouts an order at them. Suddenly one of the Frenchmen laughs. In panic fear the boy lets off the gun. It jerks in his hand; I can feel it jerking. The gun has become part of him, as though the bullets spurting out of it were a physical release from unbearable tension. . . .

"The body of the last man to fall is gaping open, as though it had been cleft with an axe instead of by bullets. The German boy is whimpering like a dog in pain. Three of the prisoners are dead, but the youngest is trying to crawl away, dragging himself along on his elbows. Both his legs are broken. The boy turns the gun on him but does not fire it. Perhaps there are no more bullets. . . .

"The boy shot himself that night. He was to be court

martialed for exceeding his orders. But that was not why he killed himself .... He killed himself because he thought he was a coward—a coward who feared whispers ....

"Pray for the soul of a German who killed Frenchmen here .... Pray for the soul of a German who killed Frenchmen here. "

"Joan! Come back Joan!" Charles's urgent voice brought me back with a jerk. I sat up and saw the warder unlocking the gates to let in a party of tourists.

"I think he killed himself on the twenty-fourth of July, 1944," I said dazedly. "I am quite certain of the rest but not of the exact date because you had to stop me."

"I nearly stopped you sooner. You kept your voice down until the last sentence which you repeated three times, very loudly and in French. The warder may have overheard."

He probably had, for he stared at me until we were safely in charge of one of his colleagues and had passed beyond the steel door which was locked behind us. We were herded into a Romanesque kitchen which, had I been less abstracted, I would have noticed was similar to the one at Glastonbury. A tourist bolder than the rest withdrew a few yards to take a photograph and was sternly ordered back to our pseudo chain gang. On our way to the refectory we passed several barred gratings among the flagstones. Were convicts now suffering as had rebellious monks in underground punishment cells? These, as a contemporary records, were "damp, lit only by a narrow window that was barred: the bed a stone slab covered with mouldy straw," in which, "on a diet of bread and water they became so blanched and skeletal that they seem like spectres rising from the tomb."

"Pray for the soul of a German . . ." kept echoing in my brain, and did not cease its insistent beat until we came to the cloister where, in spite of the neglect of the garden they enclose, a fugitive peace still lingers. I felt a lightening of spirit, a strong assurance that the prisoner had been set free of his ghost.

Although I have never seen a ghost through waiting expectantly in a place alleged to be haunted, I have met them under conditions which were socially awkward. For instance, the first time I went to Trelydan to meet Charles's mother, he warned me not to mention anything remotely related to "spooks," as, at that time, she considered that anyone who claimed second-sight must be either untruthful or unbalanced.

I was dressing for dinner when my bedroom door swung slowly open, due only to it having sagged on its hinges. Coming towards me down the long corridor was an old man, wearing a snuff-coloured waistcoat and leaning heavily on a malacca cane. As I had no clothes on I pretended not to notice him, but he paused in the doorway, looking at me very intently. Then he smiled, and stumped off along the corridor to a room beyond mine.

When I went in to dinner with Charles and his mother I was mildly surprised that three, not four, places had been laid. I presumed that the old man preferred to dine alone in his upstairs study, and prattled on about such harmless topics as herbaceous borders and the prospects for the pheasant shooting. Then I began to wonder whether the old man was another of Charles's relatives or only a fellow visitor, so I steered the conversation towards him by mentioning his snuff-coloured waistcoat. I realised there was a sudden tension, so thinking they were embarrassed because he was either senile or difficult with strangers, I tried to put them at ease by saying how friendly he had seemed, and how much I looked forward to being introduced to him.

There was a long pause. Then Mrs. Beatty said in a frigid voice, "I am unlikely to be able to introduce you to my Uncle Arthur. He has been dead for twenty years."

Shortly before the flying bombs started falling on London, Charles and I spent a week's holiday at the Savoy Hotel. On our first evening we decided to dine in the grill room. It was crowded, but we had booked a table, which was so placed that the back of my chair was against one of the square pillars.

"Charles," I exclaimed, "find another table quick . . . I'm sitting on somebody's lap!"

"Can't you pretend he isn't there?" he said, waving a waiter away. "There is no other table free, and dozens of people are waiting to eat."

"No, I can't, and I'll have to do something about it. Oh, why does he have to pick on me when hundreds of people must have sat on his lap before!"

"Why lots of people?" asked Charles. "Suppose he is someone who was here yesterday and got killed in last night's air raid? Wouldn't it be natural for him to dash back to the last safe, gay place he was in? By the way, is it he or she?"

"He. And he's been here a long time—twenty or thirty years perhaps. He's sitting here alone. *Alone* is the key. He may have had hundreds of acquaintances, but he had forgotten his real friends."

The waiter came back. We ordered something that would take time to prepare and so give me a chance to help the ghost.

It is difficult to free a ghost and remain inconspicuous in a crowded restaurant. But it worked.

As water flowing down a dry ditch gradually clears it of accumulated rubbish, so did the affection I freely offered to the ghost sweep away his loneliness until he was free to remember the people he had loved.

The table where he sat alone gradually became larger, as first one friend he had forgotten and then another came back to him on the current of affection.

When there were six guests, they went away together. And I, no longer sitting on a sad stranger's lap, was free to enjoy my dinner.

As I got up to leave the table I noticed a small brass plaque on the pillar behind my chair. It read: "This table was regularly used by Charles Frohman for many years up to 1915."

When I related this story in a newspaper article many years later the editor illustrated it with a photograph of the plaque, and added the footnote, "Charles Frohman was an American theatre impresario. He was drowned in the sinking of the *Lusitania.*"

In January 1956, Charles and I went to spend a weekend with friends near Dublin. On the Sunday morning, our host, whom I will call Patrick, took us for a long, muddy walk, and on the way home announced that we were dropping in for a drink with a neighbour.

It was a large Georgian house, and as is customary in Ireland, Patrick strode into it without ringing the bell. There was no one about, and he led us into a drawing-room on the left of the front door. "Do you find this room a bit chilly?" he enquired.

And I, who had just caught sight of myself in a mirror and realised that having neither comb nor compact I could do nothing to make myself even slightly more presentable, said rather crossly, "Of course it's chilly! What else would I expect of an Irish house in midwinter?"

"Feel one of the radiators," he suggested. I did so, and flinched because it was almost too hot to touch.

"Three large, hot radiators, and a blazing fire . . . and you still think the room is cold?"

"It is the coldest room I've ever been in," said Charles. I was relieved to hear him say so, for I felt as though a jug of ice water was being poured down my back, and hoped it was not an early symptom of flu.

Then, as I moved closer to the fire, I saw an open

coffin. I stared at it in horror and then turned on Patrick, "Taking me to a wake without even warning me may be your idea of an Irish joke, but I find it excruciatingly unfunny!"

"Wake? What on earth are you talking about?"

"Isn't 'wake' the word for the Irish custom of asking the neighbours in for a farewell drink beside the corpse?"

"Take another look," said Charles mildly.

With an effort I made myself turn round. Where the coffin had been I now saw a chintz-covered sofa.

"So it was only a spook," I said. "Sorry I got muddled."

"A very solid spook," said Charles consolingly. "I spotted there was one here as soon as we came into the room. You had better take another look at it and find out what needs doing."

I did so, seeing not with my eyes but through my forehead. This may sound odd, but it is the simplest way of describing the sensation. The man I had first seen as a corpse was now standing in the corner of the room, staring at his body, which was lying in its coffin. I described him to the others.

"The cold in this room is the cold of death. He did not believe in any form of immortality . . . that is why he is still here."

"Why didn't someone come to explain to him that he was dead?" said Patrick. "It seems a bit rough on the poor chap."

"They tried, but he wouldn't listen. He didn't love anyone, not even himself. That's why he is alone. If he had loved anyone, even for a brief period, the love would have been a lifeline which would have saved him from this icy backwater. Oh, if only people would realise how dangerous it is not to love . . . ."

"Tune out . . . quick!" said Charles, who had heard someone coming down the staircase. I switched off the other wavelength with a jerk, and said, "Patrick, don't tell them what I've seen . . . they'll think I'm dotty."

But he had already left the room, and I could hear him in the hall saying gaily, "Peggy, darling, Joan has found a coffin, tenanted, in the drawing room."

I felt embarrassed, in case she was one of the people who are offended at being told their house is haunted, as though one had complained that the drains were faulty.

But Peggy took his remark as perfectly natural. "My dear, I implored Patrick to bring you here in the hope that you would see it."

By this time we were both sitting on the sofa, which seemed rather macabre. "Did you see anything else?" she enquired eagerly.

"The *person* is in the corner over there," I said.

"Of course he is! What a comfort that you can see him too! My husband . . . luckily he is away for the weekend . . . does not believe in ghosts, and it is so unrestful having to remember not to mention them. It is a nuisance having a ghost in here because it seems to make the room so icy that we hardly ever use it even in midsummer. I want to help him, but I am not sure how to set about it. Could you give me a clue?"

"You must find out what he loves. . . . Wait a minute. There is someone else here. It's a dog, a brown and white spaniel, *his* dog. The dog died before he did, and when he thought he had lost it he became even more defensive against love. But the spaniel had more faith than her master . . . . You must make him notice that she has stayed with him: seeing her will make his heart begin to thaw."

"I knew about the dog, too," said Peggy. "Our dogs were terrified of the ghost in my home in Tipperary, and used to run yelping if we tried to take them into the haunted room. But my labrador stands in that corner wagging his tail as though asking the ghost to take him for a walk. . . . I suppose he is trying to help the spaniel make her master notice them. Now that you have given me the self-confidence I needed . . . it is extraordinary how helpful it is to meet a brother-brush . . . I shall come here with my dog tonight—after everyone else has gone to bed so that I shan't be interrupted. Instead of just praying for him, as I have often done before—and so has the priest for that matter—I shall remind him of the fidelity of his spaniel. I shall talk to him gently and with love until he *feels* that he isn't alone any more."

A few days later she telephoned to me. "He is still with us," she said. "But the coffin disappeared at once, and the room is now warm and friendly. Instead of staying in there alone he wanders all over the house and garden and seems delighted to be noticed. The children see him too, but are not in the least worried by him. After meeting you they both told me that they had always known he was there, but didn't like to mention him in case I was frightened by the coffin. Considering that when I was a child I never dared to mention ghosts to the grown-ups, it was idiotic of me not to realise that my children see them, too."

"You don't mind him still being with you?" I enquired rather anxiously.

"Of course we don't." She sounded quite indignant. "He is happy with us. He needs to be among people he can love before he will be ready to move on. He is most welcome. The only people he alarms are occasional visitors who are scared when the children talk to him, and when they see our labrador playing with an invisible dog."

It is somewhat surprising to discover that one's own ghost can be seen as most convincingly solid even when one is wide awake. An example of this phenomenon, sometimes called "astral projection," concerned Charles when he was on the French Riviera in 1938. He was sharing a villa near Mentone with six other young people, and one day, having decided to go for a long walk while the others played golf, arranged to meet them at eight o'clock in a cafe opposite the Casino.

They had been waiting for him for about twenty minutes when they saw him approaching across the square, looking very dishevelled and wearing only a pair of torn khaki shorts. This surprised them, for they were to dine at a restaurant which expected its clients to be formally dressed, and Charles had told the other two men to wear dinner jackets. As Charles was striding past they stood up and waved to attract his attention. They shouted, but he took no notice, and they saw him walk briskly into the Casino. Thinking he had mistaken the rendezvous and expected to find them in the Casino bar, they followed him there, but although they searched the place thoroughly they could not find him. By now annoyed, because they thought he was deliberately avoiding them, they went off to dine and got back to the villa about midnight.

They found Charles in bed, with a badly wrenched knee and multiple cuts and bruises. He had climbed a precipice during the morning, found he could not reach the top of it because of an overhang, and when trying to climb down again had been stranded on a narrow ledge by a small landslide which had swept away the holds he had used on the way up. Below him was a sixty foot drop, and having discovered that the rock was friable, he was reluctant to trust his weight on the only fingerhold within reach, so he decided to shout until someone heard him who could fetch a rope and haul him up.

He stayed there for seven hours, shouting until he became too hoarse and too thirsty to do more than croak. He is exceedingly meticulous about keeping appointments to the minute, especially when he is to be the host, so he became increasingly anxious at the thought of his friends waiting for him. Eventually his anxiety was stronger than his caution, which is always minimal, so he decided not to wait any longer for rescue.

At the time he was seen in Mentone he was spread-eagled against the rock face. His foothold had given way and he was clinging by his fingers to a narrow crack, with the added hazard of being blinded by the sweat pouring down his forehead. Eventually his hands became cramped and he fell, to land in a resilient thornbush. But this failed to support him for more than a couple of seconds, and he rolled another fifty feet before he could start limping, and then crawling, down to the track . . . where he got a lift home on an ox-cart.

I think many people may have seen someone who had no three-dimensional reality without realising that they have done so, as our doctor's wife, whom I will call Lydia, discovered when I was living at Trelydan. I was driving home one evening when I suddenly remembered that she was in the Cottage Hospital, because the following morning she was to have a caesarian for the birth of her second child. So I took her some flowers and gossiped for a few minutes, but only about trivialities, for at that time I had only met her briefly, and as I knew she had had a rigid "religious" background I had carefully avoided mentioning my somewhat unconventional ideas.

I knew, because her husband had told me, that the birth of her first child had been hazardous. After three days in labour, she had had an emergency caesarian, which was followed by a paralytic ileus, a dangerous complication from which she nearly died. Her husband's present anxiety was increased by the fact that she was terrified of being given an anæsthetic and always suffered from violent vomiting after ether . . this was before Pentothal was in general use.

The following morning I was engaged in one of my periodic bouts of rearranging furniture. With the assistance of three gardeners I had taken a large bookcase to pieces so that it could be moved into another room, when I suddenly noticed that it was eleven o'clock.

Lydia's operation was scheduled for noon: so I thought of her intently for two or three minutes, visualising her in her hospital room, which had a French window opening on the garden. Then I asked that someone should keep a friendly eye on her, especially before and during the an aesthetic.

I did not consciously think of her again that morning, and the only slightly unusual incident was that I was startled when the luncheon gong rang, for I thought it was only half-past eleven instead of one o'clock.

That evening the doctor called at the house to thank me for being of inestimable help to his wife. He told me that at eleven o'clock he had left her alone, as although she was very agitated he felt that his presence was only making her worse. But when he came back to take her to the theatre he found her perfectly tranquil, even drowsy. Which amazed him, for she had had no pre-medication, as she reacted badly to morphia. She told him that after he had left the room, I walked into it through the French window, and had sat by her bed, chatting so entertainingly that she had forgotten to be frightened. She seemed surprised that he had not seen me as I had only just left. She said I had assured her that she would feel so sleepy before she reached the theatre that she would need very little anæsthetic, that the baby would be fine, that she would not feel even a twinge of nausea when she came round, and would have no more pain than could be fixed with a couple of aspirins.

This is exactly what happened—a benign series of events which the doctor attributed to my powers of suggestion. He even thanked me for being tactful enough to visit Lydia by way of the garden entrance, so avoiding the dragon of a matron who would have opposed my seeing her.

I had to produce several witnesses before he was convinced that my physical body had not been within four miles of the hospital. I saw Lydia several times before I told her what had actually occurred, having warned her husband not to do so prematurely. She exclaimed, "Thank goodness I didn't know you weren't solid! I should have been terrified if I'd known I was seeing a ghost!"

According to our terminology, Lydia's use of the word "ghost" was technically incorrect, for she was seeing an aspect of my integrated self which, acting independently of my physical body, had been able to condense sufficiently to appear substantial. A ghost is a dissociated fragment of a personality which has become split off from the rest, and it remains self-imprisoned in a timeless present, whilst the integrated components continue the normal process of evolution. It has only a limited amount of energy and this will eventually run down, so a modern building is far more likely to be haunted than a medieval dungeon.

So long as a ghost remains extant, it can impinge upon a subsequent personality and may be responsible for irrational fears, compulsive behaviour, or psychosomatic conditions. For instance, if the ghost had remained in the Brussels hotel, it might be causing some man or woman, who by now could be over thirty, to have an exaggerated fear of heights. Such symptoms are, in effect, the ghost's appeal to be accepted once more into the "family" of the personality, and the release of the ghost can result in the instant disappearance of a previously intractable symptom.

It seems that the essential factor in releasing a ghost is to identify with it sufficiently to understand its particular needs. This need can be extraordinarily specific, as I learned through Old Morgan while I was still living at Trelydan.

Old Morgan, so-called to distinguish him from Young Morgan, who was a mere stripling in his seventies, had a cottage near the Top Lodge. At the age of ninety-three he developed dropsy, and was so indignant at the prospect of being bedridden that the doctor threatened to send him to hospital unless he allowed himself to be nursed instead of crawling downstairs. His sisters could not keep him in order, so Charles and I took over the job of keeping him in bed and amused during his waking hours; which was a long day as he woke with the roosters. Although that July was exceptionally hot and his bedroom stifling, he refused to let us open the window because, although he was accustomed to working outdoors in the hardest weather, he believed that fresh air when breathed between four walls was virtually lethal.

We managed to keep him cheerful, and in fact he frequently remarked that his deathbed was proving the finest holiday he had ever enjoyed. When, on the fourteenth day, he asked for another noggin of the brandy with which we kept him, and ourselves, copiously supplied, he raised his glass and gave us a most moving valedictory toast. Then he lay back on his pillows so serenely that it was several minutes before we realised he had died.

As he had taken a most sportive view of the joys awaiting him in heaven, I was dismayed when I woke the following morning and knew I had been in the churchyard where Old Morgan was lying placidly in his open grave. It was not a six-foot trench, but a shallow depression lined with finest bowling-green turf with the end curved to provide a comfortable headrest. I presumed that he was determined not to miss his funeral, but as it was not scheduled to take place until three days later, I told him to get up. To this he replied emphatically, "This is my grave, Mrs. Charles, and in it I shall lie until the Last Trump."

This was a hazard which I had not envisaged, for although he went to church every Sunday, he had seemed free of the dogmatic beliefs which can land the newly dead in difficulties. So on the following night when, in spite of my best persuasions, he remained obdurate, I left him while I achieved a convincing semblance of the conventional angel, complete with wings, white draperies, and a madonna lily. This apparition caused him to peer over the side of his grassy trough, but seeing that none of the other graves showed any sign of disturbance he declared, "I am not going to cheat my friends by going to heaven before it is officially declared open."

I cannot remember why I then found myself in the guise of a young woman, wearing an Edwardian dress and tightly corseted. Carrying a parasol in one hand and a basket of roses in the other, I heard myself saying, in a kindly but peremptory tone, "Morgan, get out of that grave immediately! It is quite ridiculous to stay there another instant, for I require you to help me with my gardens."

With a smile of ineffable joy he exclaimed, "Very good, Your Grace," and sprang lithely to his feet.

I found myself, still the Edwardian lady, standing with him on a rustic bridge which spanned a stream alight with water-lilies. His delight at the height of the rhododendrons and azaleas, the profluence of primulas, the profusion of water-loving plants beside the lake, showed me that he had known them when they were planted to translate a dream into reality. I remember seeing the great yews clipped into masterpieces of topiary, roses and yet more roses, swathes of lawn and leaping fountains. Suddenly he noticed that each flower, each leaf, even each blade of grass was in its perfection. It was then that he exclaimed, "I am in heaven!"

Through discrete questioning of Morgan's sister Jemimah, I learned that his ideal of womanhood had been the Duchess of N., for whom he had worked as a very junior member of a team of thirty gardeners during his early twenties. Jemimah looked at me very straitly with her penetrating grey eyes and said, "Morgan made a vow when he was only a boy that he would not enter heaven, even if St. Peter himself opened the Gates, until the Duchess told him to come in."

10

RAY
by Denys Kelsey

We met Ray in 1959 when she was thirty-two, and soon afterwards she asked me to see if she could learn to induce a state of auto-hypnosis so that she could use it to switch off discomforts during the later stages of pregnancy, and pain during the birth of her third child. She proved to be an excellent subject and acquired considerable proficiency in the technique in half a dozen sessions. She was in complete sympathy with our ideas and became a close friend and staunch ally. She did not live in London, and as she was fully occupied in coping, extremely efficiently, with three children, the chores of a household in which there was a constant stream of visitors, and an antique shop, we did not see her nearly as often as we would certainly have done had we all been less busy. After we moved to Collonges, in 1963, she was able to spend two short holidays with us, and we met three or four times during our infrequent visits to England.

We had not heard from her for six months when, on the sixth of June, 1966, she telephoned us. She was in a London hospital, and had just been told that a lump in her right breast had proved to be a cancer of a very malignant type and that a mastectomy would be use-

214

less. The specialist had said frankly that she had only a fifty-fifty chance of surviving for five years, though if she achieved this, the likelihood of a recurrence would each year diminish.

An indication of Ray's quality is that she spoke as though this appalling news were no more than a tiresome problem to be overcome with the minimum of trouble to anyone else. She was to have a six weeks' course of deep X-ray therapy, but this would give her an excuse to leave the chores to other people while she came to Collonges to convalesce.

She made no secret of the fact that she had cancer; but she maintained a cheerful façade to everyone except Joan, from whom she knew it was needless to conceal her real feelings. They did not often write or telephone to each other, but Joan was often with her when they were asleep. If I had had any doubts about their ability to communicate in this way, these would have been abolished by an incident which occurred on the eighth of July. Joan woke in tears, saying that Ray was feeling terribly depressed. "She is revolted by a new symptom and feels that instead of the cancer being just a lump in her breast it is spreading all over her. And what makes it even worse is that she is so *ashamed* of being in despair."

Although we knew that telephone conversations with Ray were limited to trivialities, for she was afraid of being overheard at her end of the line and causing anxiety, Joan rang up that morning, fortunately at a moment when Ray could speak freely because she was alone in the house. I picked up the extension, expecting to take part in the conversation and heard Ray describing what Joan had already told me two hours earlier. The new symptom was profuse weeping from the skin burn caused by the final dose of X-rays, a factor which cannot always be avoided in a necessarily intensive course of this treatment.

I heard Ray say, "Until the burn went so disgustingly

215

soggy and sore, I had managed to dissociate myself from the cancer, almost as though I were one of the doctors to whom I am only 'a right breast with a secondary in the armpit': now I feel it is spreading all over me. I am so ashamed of this panic! I know you are with me most nights, but tonight be even more than usually solid and give me a brisk bounce if you think there is any danger of the stiff upper lip beginning to quiver."

Ray arrived at Collonges in the late evening of the twenty-sixth of July, overjoyed to see us and not unduly exhausted, considering that she had had to leave her home three hours before taking off for Bordeaux, our nearest airport, and then had four more hours by road in ambulance.

She slept well and the following morning I made a careful physical examination. The X-rays had caused discolouration of the skin on the right side of her chest, from the base of her neck to the waist. In many places this had already started to peel and several sites were weeping profusely. The practice with hypnosis which Ray had had when we first met proved useful, for I was quickly able to induce a surgical degree of anæsthesia which meant that not only were her dressings changed without discomfort but she could immediately use her right arm freely, which she had been unable to do for several weeks. The growth was readily discernible, but there was every reason to believe that the X-rays had rendered it inactive, and I was unable to find any signs of spread. The only ominous feature, which I did not mention either to her or to Joan, was that the timbre of her voice had altered, a change undetectable when she had been speaking on the telephone, and which might be due to an enlargement of glands in her chest.

She was very optimistic about her chances of making a good recovery, an optimism which was increased by the rapidity with which her skin healed, and by the improvement in her sleep, appetite, energy, and gen-

216

eral well-being. But she took the realistic attitude that her cure was by no means certain and that she should use this opportunity to resolve any character traits which might cause her to precipitate herself back into incarnation. Or, to use her own words, "Whether I die next year or when I'm ninety, I want to be sure I shan't promptly land myself back to bawl in another pram!"

She asked us to help her to get rid of three facets of her personality. First, there was a compulsion to undertake a load of "good works" that was far larger than she could cope with; second, she had a fear that she was a coward, which often drove her to appear excessively brave; third, she had a fund of fury which she could contain only by concealing even fully justified anger. I anticipated that these would all be resolved without going beyond the framework of her current life. The first indication that in this I was mistaken occurred during our second session.

This began with her telling me that she had had a dream which had reminded her of the guilt and inadequacy she had felt at being unable to bring herself to chat to the other patients who were waiting for their turn in the X-ray unit. In the dream she had seen herself surrounded by people who, quite unlike those she had seen in the hospital, were maimed and deformed. The most distressing feature of the dream had been a feeling of intense guilt that she had been unable to change the expression of mute despair in their eyes.

I hypnotised her and asked, "From what disease were these people suffering?"

The answer came immediately: "Leprosy."

Before I could ask another question, Joan opened the door. Instead of quietly withdrawing as she would normally have done if she had inadvertently interrupted a session, she beckoned me out of the room. She told me that she had had a sudden hunch that Ray was about to tune in to a life that was concerned with leprosy. "I had a glimpse of it in a dream two nights

217

before she arrived but it was not clear enough to tell you about. It will be too tiring for her to relive it, so I will do it this afternoon and try to defuse it for her. Keep her with you while I am working in case she picks up a resonance."

Ray was surprised and even rather indignant when I parried her suggestion that we should have another session after lunch to explore the implications of her exclamation "Leprosy." But I kept her attention firmly rivetted in the present by playing Tom Lehrer on the record player.

At about five o'clock I saw Joan walking back to the house, looking very weary. She told me that she had managed to make a very close identification with an earlier personality of Ray which had been involved with lepers, in either the eighth or the ninth century A.D. This woman, who had long flaxen hair, had committed some "sin" of which the details were not entirely clear because she had accepted forgiveness for it, although only at the price of a penance. This penance had been self-inflicted and not undertaken at the command of any ecclesiastical authority. The "sin" was connected with the death of the woman's husband, who had been killed—probably murdered when it was recognised that he had contracted leprosy during a long absence abroad. The region where she lived was forested with pine trees and the people had fair skins, so it may have been Sweden or one of the other Baltic countries.

The woman, for nine years, had made herself responsible for the care of the lepers. She provided them with shelter, in wooden huts built in a forest clearing. She took them food, dressed their wounds, and—in her eyes by far the most important service— brought them the Bread of the Eucharist, for they were not permitted even to approach the chapel. Joan recalled many terrible details about the condition of each patient, of whom there were between fifty-five and sixty—she could not be more precise:

details which I was thankful Ray had not had to see.

Then this woman herself had contracted leprosy. She knew this only when, carrying a rush light which had burned so low that it was singeing her hand, the priest, instead of giving her the Bread, stared at her in horror and then fled through a door behind the altar. He must have known that total insensitivity of the fingers is one of the early signs of this disease. The woman also fled, alone into the forest. There, consumed with remorse at no longer having the courage to look after the people who trusted her, she died. Joan was not sure whether she died from cold—it was winter—or whether she carried out her intention of hanging herself with her belt.

I told Ray only the bare outlines of this story, but it was sufficient for her to accept its validity. She said she felt as though a tremendous burden had been lifted from her shoulders: and I had never seen her so gay and carefree as she was that evening.

During luncheon a few days later, when the complement of guests and children had been augmented by four others who had arrived unannounced with books for Joan to sign, I noticed that Ray was unusually silent. When people had dispersed, some to swim in the Dordogne, others to go with Joan to see a chateau, she marched determinedly to my study.

The door had hardly closed behind us when she exploded, "You must find out where my rage comes from! It flares up when I least expect it. One of the droppers-in whom Joan insisted on feeding made a fatuous remark about our lovely village. I just managed not to make a riposte which would have sent her scuttling in shame for her silliness, but I was so choked with fury that I couldn't eat anything and she went on placidly munching!"

I calmed her down and then induced hypnosis. At the count of "ten" I asked her what word came into her mind. The word was "Stone."

It occurred to me that this might be leading to a scene in which she had been stoned to death, and I was considering whether it would be better to break off the session until Joan had returned, when Ray continued, "I can see a stone wall. It is wet. I am in a cell . . . the light comes through a circular opening above me. About seven feet from the ground there is an iron ring in the wall . . ."

At this point she became very distressed and asked me to bring her back to the present. But when I had done so, instead of accepting my suggestion that we should postpone any further exploration, she said "The scene is still too vivid and I know I must go through with it."

When she had again shifted level I asked her how she got into the cell. "I am being dragged there by an infuriated mob. I can see their feet . . . filthy and ragged. I am a man . . . I wear a brown robe like a monk's habit.... How *dare* they do this to me!"

She paused and then said urgently, "Count up to twenty and get me out further . . . I must see *why* they are doing this to me . . ."

I had only begun to count when she exclaimed, "It is because of what I was doing with the acolytes!" She sounded astonished. "I only did it because I was *so bored!* I was bored with everyone in that horrible little community . . . they are poor and mean and degraded . . . even the countryside is hideous . . . hot and dusty and barren: not a tree in sight . . . only a few goats. Every day three men come into the cell and tie me by my arms to the ring in the wall . . . they leave me hanging there while the people look down through the hole above me and jeer. The wall is so smooth that I cannot get any purchase on it with my feet to ease the agony in my shoulders. Oh God how I hate them! Hate them even more than they hate me!"

As I still thought it possible that she had been stoned to death, I asked, "Did the people throw anything?"

220

"No. They only jeered . . . and at last they no longer bothered even to torment me . . . no one came to my cell . . . I had no water, and no food . . ."

"Did you stay there to haunt them?"

"I hope so! It would have served them bloody well right!"

This was said with such gusto that I had no doubt that it was the desire for revenge which had caused a fragment of that personality to become anchored in the cell. I thought we could discuss the implications of this attitude better in normal consciousness, so I brought her out of hypnosis.

She recognised that she had found the reservoir of rage which had seemed about to break its barriers whenever she felt that she, or someone of whom she was fond, was being misjudged or even slighted. She recognised also that the cause of the man in the cell becoming a ghost had nothing to do with the actions which had led to his persecution, but was solely his hatred and his desire for revenge.

For an hour or more I reminded her of various episodes in current life about which, in spite of several sessions directed towards trying to show her that they were irrelevant, she had continued to feel extremely resentful. Now she could see them impartially, from the other person's point of view as well as from her own, and made such comments as, "It wasn't his fault—I was deliberately being tiresome," or "I drooled with sympathy because I was frightened of being cross, when what would have done far more good was a brisk bounce."

Then she was silent for several minutes, until she exclaimed, "At last I can see how loathesome it is to bear grudges! I am free! Goodness I feel so happy!"

Even when in the best of health Ray had always suffered from insomnia and, like Joan, considered it perfectly normal to read at least one book before she even tried to sleep and during the night would probably start on another. Her bedroom was next to ours and if Joan saw that her light was still on after a couple of hours she would go to see whether she wanted tea, soup, or company, or perhaps a moonlight stroll in the garden. Ray had promised to fetch Joan if she had a twinge of pain or even if she was feeling lonely: so we were both worried when she admitted that for two nights running she had lain wide awake because she was racked with sciatica.

I was relieved to find that the sciatica was coming from nothing more sinister than a patch of lumbar fibrositis. Ray was convinced that its origin was psychological, but as I wanted her to have several days rest before giving her the chance of delving into another incarnation, I tried to cure it by physical means, and with straight hypnotic suggestion. I persisted with this policy for two days, but as it proved entirely ineffective I hypnotised her and asked for a clue which might lead us to its real source.

After a long pause she said, "Saddle." Then, without further prompting, "It has a high back and the stirrups are of leather, not iron. I am swaying in the saddle, for I have been riding a very long time. I am terribly tired . . . . So is the horse . . . it can hardly stand up. I am wearing some sort of armour and a tunic, but am bareheaded. My left leg is hanging down useless . . .not in the stirrup . . . I can't move it. I cannot see what I am wearing on my leg . . . it is not chainmail . . . a sort of spiral armour. My knee is very swollen and I cannot get the armour off."

I asked her if she were feeling pain anywhere else. She was silent for two or three minutes and then said, "I seem to have hurt my head . . . here," pointing to her right temple. I asked her to see how her leg was injured.

"There was a great commotion . . . many people, many horses. I cannot see what weapon I am fighting with . . . I think it is a sword. Others have swords, some only staves . . . they are on foot. I have fallen off my horse. I was heaved off it by someone on foot . . . it was then that my knee was crushed. It was not a formal battle . . . we were a party making our way to the sea to embark on boats."

"How did you come to be alone?"

"I don't know . . . someone must have put me on the horse—I could not have mounted by myself . . . . It is not my own horse! My leg is terribly painful and so is my back. I know I am bound to die. I must stay on the horse. . . a lot of blood . . . on the sand . . . all over the ground . . . but it is not mine . . ."

"Were any of your friends killed?"

"All of them, I think. There is only me left." Then, in a very subdued voice, "I left someone there . . . He is on the ground. I kept saying to myself 'He will die in a moment.' I took his horse. I should have stayed with him . . . I shouldn't have gone. I got on the horse by levering myself up from a rock, and fled out of sheer fright. I should have stayed there . . . he was still conscious. I can never forgive myself for deserting him..."

It was obvious that she was in an anguish of remorse, so I tried to comfort her by saying, "If it had been you who was deserted, would you have found it impossible to forgive him?"

"Of course not! It would not even have been difficult."

"Then why do you imagine that his capacity for forgiveness is so much smaller than your own?"

"I don't! Of course I don't! He was a far braver and more generous man than I . . . that is why I cannot forgive myself for leaving him . . ."

"Then he must long ago have forgiven you: why will you not use his forgiveness to forgive yourself!"

She was silent for several minutes. "Through false pride. I was too arrogant to accept forgiveness for being a coward. Cowardice was humiliating enough, and my pride made forgiveness seem a further humiliation . . . to accept it would have put me under an obligation . . . so it was easier to punish myself . . . to punish myself over and over again by trying to forget my cowardice through enduring pain I need not have suffered. But I am no longer too arrogant to accept forgiveness . . . I shall be able to forgive other people so easily, now that I can forgive myself."

After a long pause, during which she looked drawn and tense, her face relaxed into a smile of contentment. "That is over now. I am at peace with myself . . . and the difference in my leg is indescribable."

Ray left Collonges on the sixth of September, for although her appointment with the cancer specialist was not until the following week, she wanted to be home in time for the birthday of her elder son. The clinical notes I made on the previous evening read: "Her general condition is good and her morale high. The lump in the breast seems definitely smaller and is less firmly attached both to the skin and the underlying muscle. Apart from a doubtful epitrochlear gland I can find no evidence of metastases. The ominous signs are that she has lost seven pounds during the six weeks she has been here. I hope this is due only to the fact that our diet is high in protein and non-fattening. She now weighs a hundred and thirty-three pounds, a reasonable weight for a woman of five-foot eight. She gets breathless very easily during a walk, even considering that most of the tracks are steep and stony. She has less stamina than I should have liked to see and there is still that change in the timbre of her voice. We can only hope that these signs do not indicate a persistence of the cancer process."

As Ray telephoned to assure us that she had not been unduly tired by the journey and that her household was running so smoothly that she could continue to give herself every chance further to recuperate, Joan and I seized the opportunity of a gap between batches of visitors to go to Paris, where we intended to stay for a week.

On the thirteenth Ray telephoned, having just got home from seeing the specialist. "The lump in my breast is inactive so that's fine," she said. Then she added, "But I noticed several little pea-sized nodules in my scalp yesterday and another on my forehead. It seems that these are very glum news. He says there are also secondary deposits in my left arm and in the wall of my chest."

Joan and I were so distressed by these new signs that it was futile to pretend that we could enjoy a holiday, so we came home the following morning. Ray's physician, Peter, with whom I had often corresponded though not yet met, telephoned on the seventeenth to say that he believed her prognosis to be very gloomy and that although she wished to come back immediately to Collonges, he felt that the potential medical and surgical requirements made it essential for her to remain in England. He knew that she would be bitterly disappointed at not being allowed to return to us and was wondering how best to tell her that this was inadvisable. After a hasty conference with Joan, I rang back to say that we would leave sundry visitors to look after themselves and be with Ray on the following Saturday.

We went to England by car, as we were going to stay with friends who lived about an hour's drive from Ray, to spare her the additional housekeeping problems which she would insist on undertaking if we were her guests. Joan is usually able to quell such activities with a brisk "Leave it all to me!"; but Ray, as she often ruefully admitted, found it as difficult as Joan does to sit back and let someone else do the chores, especially in her own house.

When Ray ran across the lawn to welcome us, she seemed so full of vitality, and chatted so gaily during lunch, that it was difficult to accept that the "millet-seeds" which had appeared in the lymphatics of her arms and neck, the nodules in her scalp, and the cough which was due to the rapidly enlarging glands in her chest could really be of such serious import. The specialist had told her that he wished to see her again in three weeks, when he would decide whether to remove her ovaries, or her supra-renals, or to sever the stalk of her pituitary gland—procedures which he then thought might extend her life.

Ray had accepted the likelihood of an operation and wanted it performed as soon as possible. Peter and I managed to conceal our doubts that she would ever be strong enough to undergo it.

The following day she seemed more frail, but she insisted that this was only because, after we had left, some friends had dropped in unexpectedly and she had sat up talking with them until midnight. She came downstairs about noon, and although she tried to make light of her cough it was obviously more troublesome, sometimes leading to a laryngeal spasm. However, before we left she was settled comfortably in bed and seemed confident of having a good night's sleep.

During our drive, which was prolonged from one hour to nearly three by fog and Sunday-night traffic, I asked Joan whether she thought Ray was still clinging to the hope of becoming well enough to travel out to us.

"Only with the surface of her mind—the bit she uses to conceal her feelings when she thinks they should be hidden. When we were in the garden this afternoon she told me she had dreamed of the hand again—the hand she saw stretched out to help her to cross a little river. She knew that if she clasped the hand she would not come back to her body. She first had this dream on the night she was told she had cancer, and she has had it twice since she came home. It is interesting how dying usually seems like crossing a river—I remember doing it often myself."

About half an hour later, Joan announced that she was getting "echo-symptoms" from Ray, who she felt sure was having difficulty with her breathing. I had had far too many checks on the validity of Joan's ability to resonate to other peoples' symptoms to be able to comfort myself with the hope that this was due only to anxiety. By the time we arrived Joan sounded as though she were suffering from asthma, so I was glad there was no telephone message awaiting us, for the fog was by now so thick that the return journey would have taken most of the night.

In the morning I was backing the car out of the garage when Joan came out of the house carrying an overnight bag. She slung it on the back seat saying, "We shall need this because we shan't be coming back here tonight.... I wish I had had the hunch sooner for then I would have had time to pack a suitcase."

Before I could comment we heard the telephone ringing. It was Peter, saying that Ray had suddenly had a massive collapse of her left lung and that her heart was very irregular . . . he was arranging for her immediate admission to hospital . . . she would like us to come as quickly as possible.

When we got to Ray her heart was settling down and her breathing was under control, but she said, "I have been whooping until I retched . . . worse than when I caught the children's whooping cough." She succeeded in remaining so calm and even cheerful that the young ambulance men obviously thought she was suffering from a trivial ailment and treated her in a jocular manner, intending to inspire confidence. On the way to the hospital one of them asked her, "What's the trouble? A pain in your tum?" In a moment of exasperation she replied:

"A teeny bit more tiresome than that—I'm riddled with cancer." When Ray told us this she added regretfully, "The poor boy blanched with horror and I felt such a bitch."

X-rays showed not only that her left lung had collapsed but that fluid was accumulating on the right side also. In addition she had a huge effusion, caused by cancer nodules, in the pericardium—the sac which contains the heart. There was no longer any question of operating: it was doubtful if she could even have survived the anæsthetic.

When Peter told her of this decision she realised at once that the prognosis was hopeless, and thanked him fervently for having had the kindness and the moral courage to spare her from the farce of trying to pretend that she did not know she was dying. We were equally grateful to him, and our gratitude and affection were to increase each time we met, for many doctors would have been shocked to hear us discuss death frankly with the patient.

"The sooner I die the better," Ray said forthrightly when Peter had left the room. "So you and Joan must remind me how to cross the river. I must have done it dozens of times before so I expect I shall find it quite familiar. To start with I must get out of hospital, for there are far too many interruptions—nannies popping in and out with cups of tea and the thermometers—to have a chance even to sleep—much less to practise dying."

Before we left her, late that evening, hypnosis had relieved much of her discomfort; her heart was beating quietly and regularly, her breathing was smooth. She was in such a profound sleep that I thought she might slip away during the night.

We took a room in a hotel near the hospital so that we could be with her even sooner than the twenty minutes it would have taken to drive from the house in her village where we were staying. Joan went up to have a bath while I made sure that the night porter knew our room number in case of an emergency call.

When I joined Joan she told me, with the conviction to which I am now accustomed and only rarely find irritating, "You needn't wait for the telephone to ring. Ray won't die for at least ten days. I know she could have a fatal heart attack at any minute . . . but she won't. How do I know? Because she told me this afternoon that she has decided not to die until she has made sure that the children understand what is happening, and realise that she can talk to them when they are asleep. She also wants to see various friends, especially those who she knows are scared of dying, and to tidy up her papers and give away her things. She says she felt exactly the same urge to leave everything in order when she was preparing for the birth of a baby."

The next morning Ray told us that she had slept very well and knew that she was not going to die yet because she had again dreamed of the river and it was much wider. "Instead of it being so narrow that I could easily jump across it the banks have become reedy and muddy. The only time I get scared is when I think I might get stuck in the mud. Can you promise this won't happen?"

We both gave her our most heartfelt assurance that when she decided that she wanted to discard her body she should have every assistance she needed. Joan then again told her the technique she must practice. This was to shift level, which I could help her to do with hypnosis, and then visualise herself crossing the river, each time leaving a little more of her vital energies on the far bank. "Remember that there is nothing you can do on this side that you cannot do much better on the other. You enjoy skiing—so while you are asleep this afternoon, think of the finest ski slopes you have ever seen, and you will probably wake up knowing that you have been skiing better and faster than you ever dared to imagine."

When we came back, after Ray had slept, she told us, "It worked beautifully! I skied so much better than I've ever done down here—splendid fast christies, and I went soaring over some jumps."

She stayed in hospital another two days so as to have the pericardial effusion tapped, which, although the sac would soon fill up again, caused a temporary improvement. At her suggestion, a hospital bed, which would make nursing her more easy, was put into the drawing room from which she could look into the garden through the three French windows. Friends who arrived at the house, apprehensive at the thought of talking to a woman who they knew was dying, relaxed within a couple of minutes, and were soon talking freely, laughing, drinking whisky or sharing Ray's champagne, as though nothing could be more natural than that she should be discussing her imminent departure to a country to which she longed to return.

It was decided not to repeat the tapping of the pericardium because sudden cardiac arrest would be preferable to the respiratory failure which could not be long delayed, for by now only the tip of her remaining lung was functioning. Yet she continued to laugh and talk and read, to sort out the papers which crammed the drawers of two desks, to dictate letters. She decided to have a memorial service, "which will give my friends a chance to meet each other"; and left instructions for her body to be cremated, "with no one there except the professionals." A river flows through her village, and she wished her ashes to be scattered from the bridge.

Although her physical reserves were so slight that it was an effort to reach for a glass or a powder compact from the table beside her bed, her peace of mind made the control of her symptoms by hypnosis so effective that she required only minimal doses of analgesic drugs, an occasional tablet of codeine to control a spasm of coughing, and a modest dose of a barbiturate at night. If she had a twinge of pain when I was not within call, she could switch it off by swinging a brass clock key on a piece of ribbon . . . this being the "trigger object" which I had chosen, merely because it had happened to be on the mantelpiece and was a convenient size.

Every afternoon I helped her to practice dying. I would induce the extreme depth of hypnosis and she would describe what she was seeing "on the other side of the river." She was always enchanted by the extraordinary beauty of the scenery, the lakes in which she could swim so freely under water, the mountains she climbed with such ease, the gardens in which flowers grew without being regimented by the seasons.

I asked her whether there was anything I could do to make her crossing easier. Without a second's hesitation she said, "I shall just step across. I know this is true for the river has become so narrow that it is only a little stream."

I told her to sleep, and when her breathing had changed to a slow, peaceful rhythm I left the room, for I wanted to warn Joan that I thought Ray might not wake again.

Joan had gone back to the cottage, and I found her sitting on the bed with her hands pressed to her temples. She glanced up: "Listen: this is very important. Something is going wrong inside Ray's head. I got an echo of it during lunch, which is why I bolted back here instead of going to see her. I can often manage to deflect her pain, but this head pain is so terrible that I doubt if I would be able to do anything about it."

Joan had no inkling that Peter and I had both been only too well aware that Ray might possibly develop secondaries within her skull which could cause extreme pain, and when I talked with Peter he accepted without question, as I had done, the validity of Joan's hunch. While I was talking with him, Joan was with Ray. Then she joined us and said, "Ray has told me that she knows she will stay alive as long as we are here with her. She wants us to go back to France the day after tomorrow, by the night boat. She is going to ask Peter to be with her when we leave, and stay with her until she is very far out: and then she thinks she will be able to cross the Channel with us."

"I will most certainly do so," said Peter. "And my Joan will come to her early the next morning."

Peter's wife is also called Joan, and shares his qualities: I can pay her no greater or more sincere tribute.

The next day Ray was feeling so well that she thought there must have been a mistake in the X-rays. Before I could remind her that these were confirmed by Peter's daily examination of her chest, she picked up the hand mirror and studied her lovely face attentively. "I can't really be on my deathbed when I haven't any discomfort! My hair hasn't gone dank . . . it's lucky I'm a genuine blonde or I would have gone dark at the roots by now. And my skin is all right and my nails have never looked better, even if my fingers have gone numb. I'm very wobbly if I try to stand, but who wouldn't be after being so long in bed? Do you realise it's three weeks today since they carted me off to the hospital?"

About half an hour later she suddenly gasped and clutched her side. She had an acute pain in her chest which hypnosis did not relieve. I was about to give her an injection of pethidine when Joan took Ray's hand and said, "Listen, darling: you are giving yourself this pain, to prove that there hasn't been some ghastly medical muddle. It is totally unnecessary, so switch it off at once!"

In a couple of minutes Ray relaxed and lay back on her pillows. "Thank God it has gone! A day or two of pain like that and I should be crazy!"

It was very understandable that she should have sought this assurance, for except during the moments of exhaustion evoked by any change of position, it was difficult even for Peter and me to realise that she was a dying woman.

Her only lingering anxiety had been that as no one she loved had already died, she might feel lonely; but by now she had several times remembered being with a man whom she described as "one of my special people," whom she thought she had first known when they were both Greek. She knew also that she would soon meet not only her own loves of the long years, but the people to whom Joan and I had been linked through the centuries by affection.

On the last day, she said again, "I believe that dying has been the most important thing I have done in my life, for it seems to have made so many people less frightened. I am so very glad that you have promised to hand it on by writing about me . . . and I'll try to help." Of our parting, I will say only that the three of us shared a poignant sorrow and a profound peace which I had not previously known could coexist.

I had expected that we would be conscious of Ray on the boat that night. But although I slept deeply, and Joan remained wide-awake, trying to shift level, neither of us could make contact with her.

The following morning, after we had been driving south for about two hours, we were both vividly conscious that Ray was also in the car, but the awareness faded after a few minutes. During the early afternoon, Joan, who was driving, suddenly stopped the car, saying, "Don't worry about me: I must be alone for a few minutes." She came back looking preoccupied, and said that she was not yet sure whether we should go to our favourite hotel at Chaumont, on the south bank of the Loire, or stay on the north bank, in Blois.

It was sunset when we reached the river. Again Joan stopped the car. Then she said steadily, although I knew she was close to tears, "It is all right now. We can go to Chaumont." She did not have to tell me that we could cross the Loire because Ray had already crossed her river.

As soon as we had gone up to our room we put a trunk call through to Peter. He told us that before he had given Ray an injection to ensure that she slept, she

233

had talked to him for about an hour. Her serenity, her assurance of the happiness she was so soon to find, had been the culmination of three weeks in which she had given him and his wife something of inestimable value which they would treasure all their lives. Ray had slept until late the following morning, but then woke, to say regretfully to Peter's Joan who was already with her, "I'm still here .... and I tried so hard not to come back." When Peter arrived she was having a paroxysm of coughing, so he gave her another injection. They both stayed with her while she slept, and the only time she opened her eyes it was to say, "They are waiting for me. And they are all smiling. And they have such happiness in their faces." At four-fifteen her heart stopped beating.

This confirmation brought us a joy and relief which was overwhelming; a joy shared by Ray, for suddenly she was with us, free and radiantly happy. She could hardly have been more perceptible if she had still been using a physical body.

Although I had had empirical evidence of the ease with which thoughts can be exchanged between people who are functioning on different levels of reality—as when Joan perched on my knee and dictated extremely useful material while her body was under an anæsthetic, I had assumed that Ray would help me to write about her by causing me to have flashes of insight or lucid dreams. But on the twenty-ninth of October, while I was discussing with Joan which extracts to use from my very detailed case notes, she said, "As Ray is here, why don't you ask her?"

I protested that this was her expertise rather than mine; but Joan insisted that it would be easier for Ray to get ideas through to me because of the link we had already established through the use of hypnosis.

I decided to try the technique which, as I have already mentioned, I sometimes use during a session to increase the free flow of intuition. This consists in closing my eyes, withdrawing attention from sensory stimuli, and shutting out ideas which stem only from my intellect. A patient seldom realises what I am doing, though there have been occasions when it took more than a couple of minutes and he has enquired, with solicitude or resentment, whether I have fallen asleep. As only Joan was present, I was able to increase the ease of relaxation by lying full length on the sofa; and as I knew that a level-shift which lasts for more than a few minutes is likely to produce a marked drop in body temperature, I covered my legs with a rug.

I was doubtful that I would be able to make any contact with Ray, for I had not been aware of her presence; but within seconds I knew that she was there. I signed to Joan to ask me a question.

"What does Ray wish us to write about her?"

The answer came immediately: "What *fun* it is to die! Dying is not at all solemn.... There is not even the sadness I expected at being physically parted. I can always make contact with the upstairs part of you, so for me there is no feeling of separation. It is not nearly so easy for you, because sometimes you can't remember that we have been together."

"What was dying like?"

"Just what I expected . . . crossing a river which had become so small a stream that I could literally step across it. There was no sense of strangeness, for I had been to the river so often when we were practising. There was nothing to fear because I had seen the Beautiful Country before I came back to it. You and Joan *knew* what you told me was true . . . you could not have been nearly so helpful if you had only *hoped* that it might be."

"Did remembering some of your own lives help you?"

"It only confirmed what I already knew . . . I was convinced that I had lived many times the moment you reminded me, years ago, about reincarnation . . . it seemed so obvious even then that I could not have doubted it even if I had wished to . . . There were so many people to welcome me . . . I had forgotten how many people I had loved, and still loved, even though I had not seen them for centuries . . ."

I had a clear visual impression of Ray: although my eyes were closed, I could see her sitting on the arm of the sofa. I could not hear her voice, but the communication was as clear as though words were being dictated; words which I repeated so that they would be registered by the tape recorder.

Within a few days it had become almost as natural to say, 'Why not ask Ray?" as it would have been to suggest consulting her by telephone. I could seldom keep a clear contact for more than half an hour, and when I felt unable to condense her thoughts into words without hesitation, or if my visual impression of her was becoming hazy, I told Joan to turn off the tape recorder. Sometimes my awareness of her would fade gradually: sometimes it ended as abruptly as though a television set had been switched off.

I found that contact was either established very quickly, within a couple of minutes, or that there was none at all. I have had completely negative results on about half of the occasions when I have induced a level-shift in order to ask some specific question, and on these, however hard I tried to visualise her, or to make myself believe that she was present, such efforts proved entirely ineffective.

There have been times when Joan or I, or both of us simultaneously, have realised that Ray was with us even though we had not been thinking about her for several days. For instance, we were having dinner in the buffet of Brive railway station before meeting visitors who were arriving by the Paris express, when I suddenly realised that she was sitting in the empty chair at the table. She wanted me to tell the young man who was dining with us how grateful she had been that he had driven half across England to see her before she died.

At Ray's suggestion I have included only the questions and her replies which are relevant to this book, and these occurred in the course of seven different sessions. In nearly every session she repeated, "Tell them how easy it is to die. If you can remind them that they have had many lives, they will know that there is no need to fear dying . . ."

"Why was it so easy for you to get out of your body?"

"I had no fear of shedding it. I knew it should be shed quickly, because the cancer was spreading so fast that nothing could have prevented me from feeling pain much longer.... I think Joan knew that it was starting in my head. My body would soon have become a barrier between me and the people I loved.... There is no point in keeping a body which is no longer a useful means of expressing the rest of oneself. Even two more days would have made it difficult for me to leave smoothly...."

"Why would pain have made it more difficult to die? I should have thought that pain would have made death even more welcome."

"Pain, not death, is always the enemy. Pain wastes the energy which, when it can no longer be used for healing the body, is needed to get out of it. Pain can so easily become confused with the simple little act of dying . . . there is nothing to be gained through pain . . . it is this pain, the futile suffering, which has caused so many people to fear death."

"If you had no fear of death, why did you have the X-rays?"

"Because I didn't want to leave the people I loved, especially when I was learning how to be useful . . . I had forgotten that I could be far more useful up here than I was when I had to filter everything I knew through my intellect. On this level it is so much easier to make people understand that I am trying to help them, and not just being bossy!"

"What kind of work are you doing?"

"Helping to rescue ghosts . . . and showing people how easy it is to cross the river . . . and trying to make them wake up in the morning knowing that they can stop being so silly . . ."

"If you had not rescued your ghosts before you died, would you have had to come back here to do so?"

"I *need* not have been born again . . . but I would probably have gone on refusing to acknowledge their existence while I was up here. I was too ashamed to bring them with me to this side of the river. Ghosts are very like discreditable relatives that one tries to disown . . . I could not have ignored them indefinitely, because they had to come home before I could be a whole person . . . this is difficult to translate into words . . . 'I' used to mean Ray . . . now it means all the experience, incarnate and excarnate, which adds up to what, up here, I mean when I think of myself as 'Me.'"

"Could you have freed your ghosts while you were down here unless you had been able to remember them?"

"Of course I could! They would have started to become free whenever I chose to change the direction of the energy which was keeping them imprisoned."

"So it was not essential to remember them?"

"It helped a very great deal . . . more than I think you realise. When I could no longer disown them, I knew it was too *squalid* to cling to my false pride any longer: too snobbish to pretend that they did not exist. False pride was the source of all my ghosts. I refused to admit that the people I could have helped turned against me because I despised them: I refused to admit that I looked after the lepers only because they provided me with a convenient penance: I refused to admit that I left a brave man to die in pain only because I had not the courage to set him free of his body."

"Why did you take so long to forgive your ghosts?"

238

"Before I could forgive *them,* I had to forgive *myself* . . . It was much easier to punish myself . . . but all that the self-punishing did was to feed my false pride! Self-punishing often drives people to shrive their guilt by inflicting on themselves the misery they have caused . . . and this never does anyone any good . . . it only adds to the sum of suffering. It is so sad and so *silly!*"

"Who decides whether, or when, you will come back here again?"

"Me! You both know this perfectly well! No one is ever *sent* into incarnation. We are born either because we want to be able to hide our unloveable traits from other people . . . and even from ourselves . . . or because we have volunteered to try to make the pattern come true on the downstairs level."

"Why do so few 'down-here' people know about the Beautiful Country?"

"Because they are blinded by the aspects of themselves which have never been here . . . which could not come up here because they relished rage and hatred, or wanted to continue making someone else feel small, or gloated over possessions, or believed they could own people . . . And the part of their upstairs self which has gone back to try to educate the delinquent aspects finds it difficult enough to be in exile, without remembering the contrast between up here and down there . . . remembering would make them even more homesick."

It is now the twentieth of February, 1967. I have not talked with Ray for ten days. At the close of our last session she said, "I am not going to answer any more questions until you have finished the book. I have already told you what I want you to say about me. Tell them how easy it is to cross the river . . . tell them there is no loneliness up here and so much joy to share. Hand on what we all know to be true."

We have tried to do so.

239

THE FAR MEMORIES

Ariel Press is proud to announce that it has brought all seven of Joan Grant's "far memory" novels back into print in a uniform collection of books. They may be purchased either individually or as a set. The books, and their prices, are:

Winged Pharaoh. $11.95.
Life as Carola. $9.95.
Return to Elysium. $9.95.
Eyes of Horus. $11.95.
Lord of the Horizon. $11.95.
Scarlet Feather. $10.95.
So Moses Was Born. $9.95.

These books can be purchased either at your favorite bookstore or directly from Ariel Press (include an extra $2 per book for postage; $3 for Canada and overseas).

For those who prefer, the entire set of seven novels plus Joan Grant's autobiography, *Far Memory,* (which sells by itself for $10.95), may be purchased as a subscription for $80 postpaid—a savings of $25. *No substitutions or deductions are allowed on subscriptions.*

Also available is a one-of-a-kind memoir by Joan Grant, *A Lot To Remember,* which records her physical— and supernatural—journeys through the Lot region of France. It sells for $10.95 plus $2 postage.

Copies of *Many Lifetimes* cost $12.95, plus postage.

All 10 books may be ordered for $99 postpaid.

All orders from the publisher must be accompanied by payment in full in U.S. funds. Please do not send cash. Send orders to Ariel Press, P.O. Box 1387, Alpharetta, GA 30239.

For faster service, call toll free 1-800-336-7769 and charge the order to VISA, MasterCard, Discover, Diners Club, or American Express.